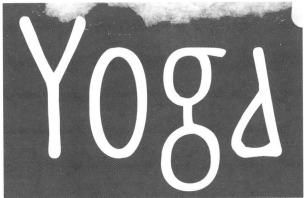

FOR IDEAL
WEIGHT AND SHAPE

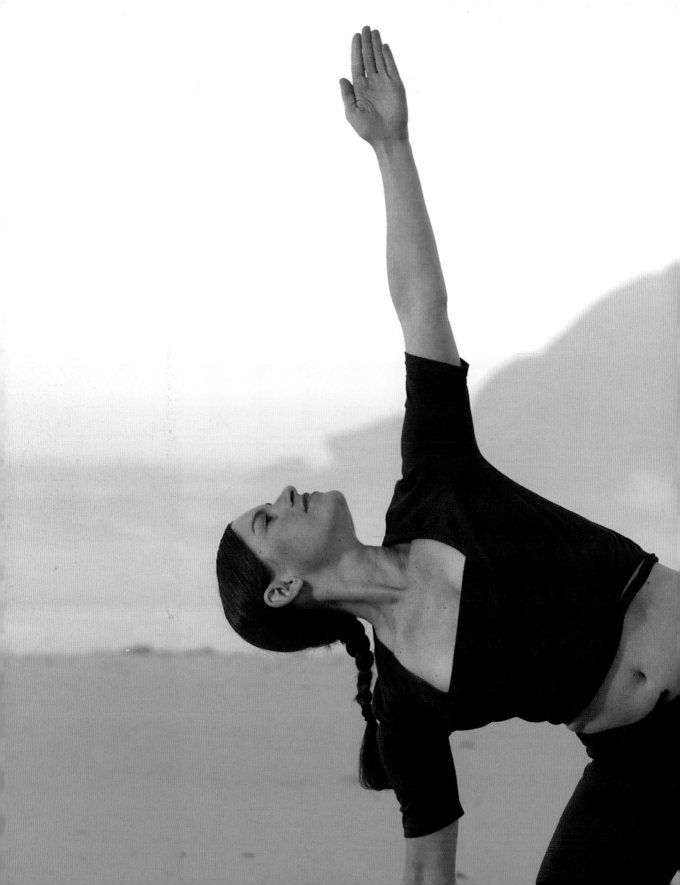

Yoga

FOR IDEAL WEIGHT AND SHAPE

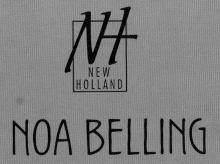

NEW
HOLLAND

NOA BELLING

First published in Australia in 2006 by
New Holland Publishers (Australia) Pty Ltd
Sydney • Auckland • London • Cape Town

14 Aquatic Drive Frenchs Forest NSW 2086 Australia
218 Lake Road Northcote Auckland New Zealand
86 Edgware Road London W2 2EA United Kingdom
80 McKenzie Street Cape Town 8001 South Africa

The National Library of Australia Cataloguing-in-Publication data:
    Belling, Noa.
    Yoga for ideal weight and shape.
    Includes index.
    ISBN 9781741102987 (hbk).
    1. Yoga. 2. Hatha yoga. I. Title.
    613.7046

ISBN(10) 174110 298 7
ISBN(13) 978 174110 298 7

Publisher: Fiona Schultz
Project Editor: Lliane Clarke
Editor: Anna Tannenberger
Designer: Maryna Beukes
Production: Monique Layt
Reproduction by Resolution Cape (Pty) Ltd
Printer: SNP/Leefung Printing Co. Ltd (China)

10 9 8 7 6 5 4 3 2 1

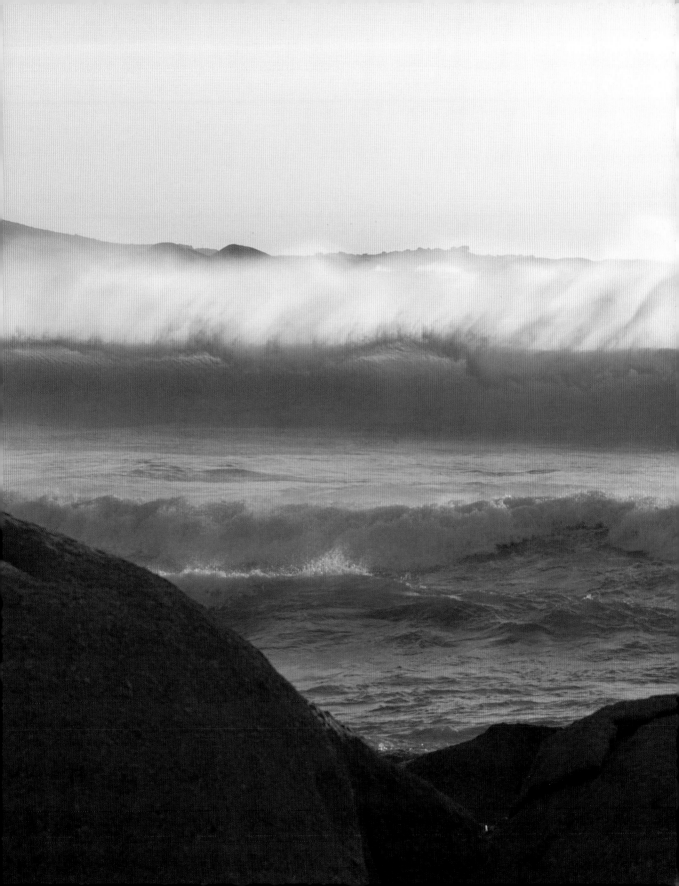

INTRODUCTION   8

1. BODY TYPES   16

2. FITNESS AND BODY TONE   22

3. THE PSYCHOLOGY OF WEIGHT LOSS   32

4. DIET AND LIFESTYLE   38

5. POSTURE INSTRUCTION   46

6. YOGA SESSIONS FOR SLIMMING AND BODY TONING   102

7. VINYASA—YOGA POSTURE FLOWS   140

8. SPECIAL CONSIDERATIONS   148

AKNOWLEDGEMENTS   150
INDEX   151

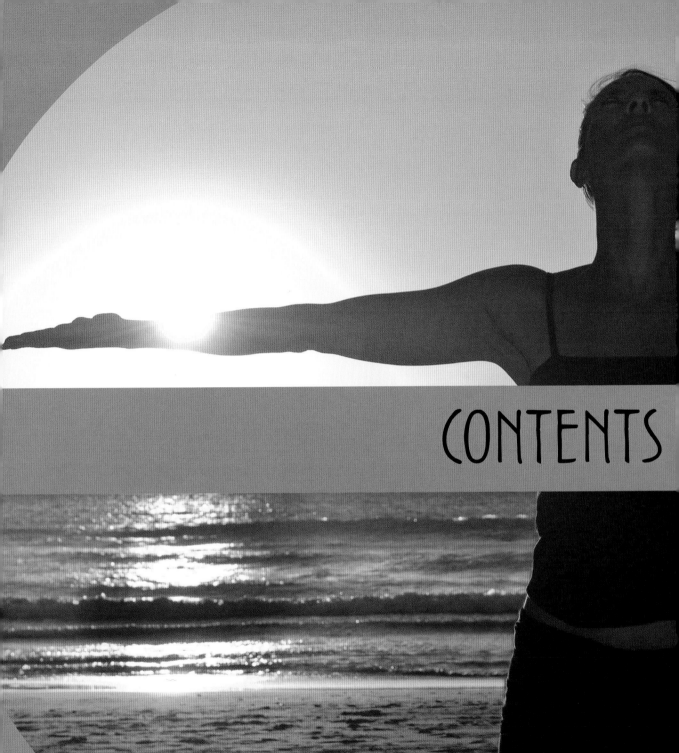

CONTENTS

A New Relationship

Yoga for Ideal Weight and Shape is a book about achieving and maintaining your ideal body weight and shape. Along with this comes a new relationship with your body. It is a journey toward better understanding your body and learning to honour and appreciate it.

It is also an empowering journey of discovering that you can influence your life in desirable ways. This book is ideal for self-practice. It is suitable for beginners and advanced practitioners, for adolescents and seniors. It is also suitable for people of varying degrees of physical fitness.

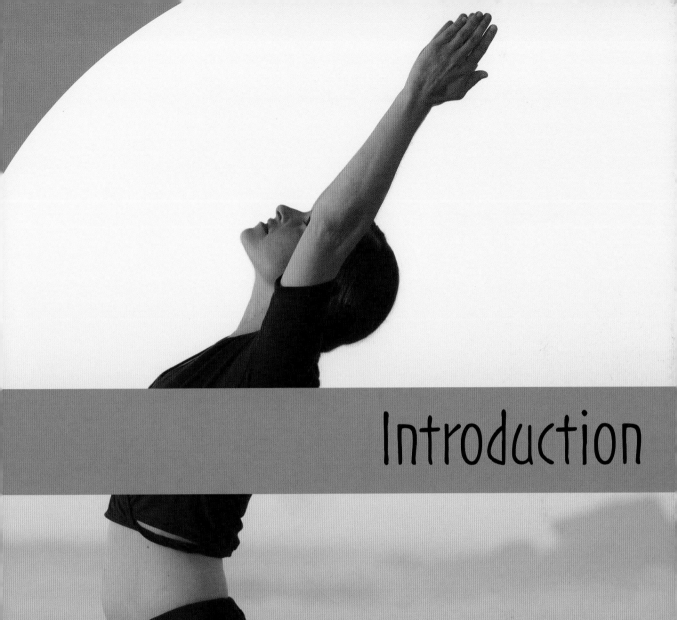

Introduction

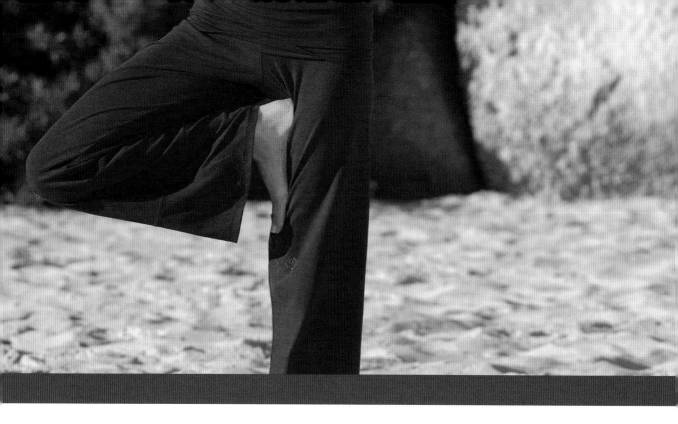

Yoga and Weight Loss

Yoga is a centuries-old system of personal development and health cultivation originating in India. Yoga is a Sanskrit word which means 'to unite' or 'to harmonise'. The essence of Yoga is the achievement of harmony, within oneself and in relation to others and one's environment.

HOLISTIC HEALTH

It is now becoming common knowledge worldwide that health is not only physical. Emotional, mental and spiritual factors also play their part. This is something the Yogis have known for centuries. Yoga provides a structure for exploring the relationship between the physical and spiritual; and encouraging the integration of these aspects. This is achieved through guidance in exercising the physical body thoroughly and, through this, deepening awareness of the emotional and spiritual dimensions of your life.

YOGIC VIEW ON BODY WEIGHT

Body weight is a physical expression of good health. Conversely, the condition of being over or underweight is viewed as one of many signs of imbalance or 'dis-ease' in the human system. The cause of overweight is generally attributed to lifestyle choices, which in turn are influenced by physical and psychological factors. For this reason, achieving an ideal weight is essentially a process of recovering health. And for this ideal weight to be sustainable, the process of recovery needs to take physical and psychological factors into account.

Two ways to view weight loss

The topic of weight loss can be viewed from two angles: what you lose; and what you gain. The first is a consideration of what you are moving away from; the second on what you are moving toward. The main focus of this book is on what you gain. It is the more inspiring option, with Yoga as supportive tool.

What you lose

On a physical level, losing weight leads to:
- » *Losing excess fatty tissue, which can be measured in centimetres around the areas of your body where there has been fat accumulation.*
- » *'Losing' poor health that resulted from sluggish functioning of body systems, such as blood and lymph circulation and digestion.*
- » *'Losing' low energy levels. When body systems are not functioning optimally, they require more energy to carry out normal physiological processes. This robs us of energy that could be available for daily functioning. Excess fatty tissue also makes the body heavier than it needs to be, requiring more energy for movement and carrying out daily tasks.*
- » *'Losing' poor muscle tone and inflexibility.*

On a psychological level, losing weight can lead to:
- » *'Losing' low self-esteem and depression.*
- » *'Losing' the dislike of your own body; and lack of self-confidence.*
- » *'Losing' the inability to trust yourself; of feeling that your appetite and your life are out of control.*
- » *'Losing' a physical shape of which you are not proud.*
- » *'Losing' any number of other self-deprecating psychological attitudes that come with feeling overweight.*

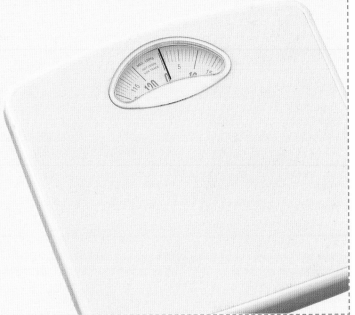

WHAT YOU GAIN

From a holistic perspective you can:

» *Gain a slimness that is appropriate for you.*
» *Gain health and vitality through improved body system functioning.*
» *Gain increased energy levels.*
» *Gain a body that is more resilient and less prone to injury.*
» *Gain a state of being where energy efficiency, mental clarity, emotional resilience and a playful spirit weave together to inform and guide your experience of life.*
» *Gain a body shape about which you feel good. This involves feeling at home in your body; that it is a welcome part of you.*
» *Gain your beauty and sensuality. Sensuality is about engaging with the world more fully and satisfyingly through all your senses, including the enhanced ability to tune in to the feelings and sensations of your body. Yoga is an ancient, classic system for training such body awareness.*

Enhanced sensuality can also lead to more fulfilling sexuality.

» *Gain improved skin tone with a healthy glow to your skin from improved circulation. This, together with improved health and body tone, can reduce and delay the physical signs of ageing.*
» *Gain self-discipline, self-confidence and self-respect.*
» *Gain mastery over your appetite, which is one of the most challenging conquests for the human being. This is especially true in these times of excess supply and commercial temptation. Appetite can refer to any form of indulgence. While a good appetite is inherently healthy, becoming a slave to one's appetites can lead to greed, imbalance and ill-health. Applying a daily discipline, including healthy eating and a physical practice such as Yoga, can greatly assist in the challenge of taming temptation.*

WHEN WEIGHT LOSS MAY BE UNHEALTHY

There are people who struggle to gain weight, or at times may lose excessive amounts of weight unintentionally. Both can be signs of imbalance or ill-health. The Yoga practices offered in this book can also benefit these people by cultivating health and toning the body systems involved in regulating and maintaining healthy body weight.

In the case of an Eating Disorder, where a person may intentionally lose more weight than is healthy, this book can also be a valuable tool with which to increase body awareness. Yoga practice also promotes a healthy relationship with your appetite and

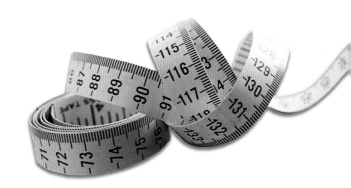

eating patterns, while encouraging a kind and caring attitude towards your body and, by extension, your experience of life.

IDEAL WEIGHT, IDEAL SHAPE

What is ideal weight? How can you tell whether or not you are at your ideal weight? And is your ideal weight realistic for your body type or based on some unattainable ideal flaunted in fashion magazines? Is your image of ideal weight more about an ideal shape—one which may not have any bearing to the actual shape of the body you were born into?

Is ideal weight or shape a personal, inner-referenced experience, or something determined from outside yourself? Is it something you can feel or is it based on the opinion of others, or cultural, societal ideals, or tables that tell you what your ideal weight should be in relation to your height, weight or fat percentage?

Yoga is a training ground for inner-referenced awareness, starting in Hatha Yoga, with attention to the body in postures, and moving beyond this to naturally meeting your attitudes toward yourself and your life. For this reason, from a Yogic perspective, ideal weight is not seen as a specific, measurable number or amount relative to height, age or fat percentage, or any other means of determining your weight from a source outside yourself. This would mean deeming outside sources as experts over and above yourself, with these outer sources determining what is acceptable for you and your body. This is disempowering because it robs you of the opportunity to exercise your inner knowledge; your inner wisdom. Yoga is all about cultivating your internal evaluation and motivation system, based on how you feel and what you deem appropriate and desirable. Added to this is an inner strength and willpower generated through Yoga practice.

In Yoga ideal body weight and shape are considered natural byproducts of health. For this reason, the question of what is ideal body weight naturally leads to a broader question of what is health and how to cultivate it. The order of importance in the process of moving toward ideal weight is health first, which deter-

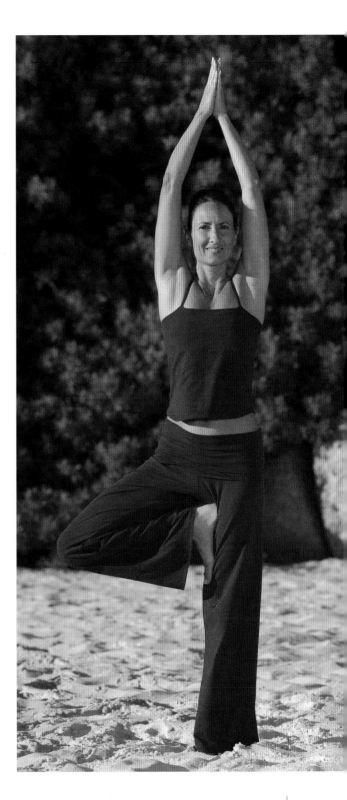

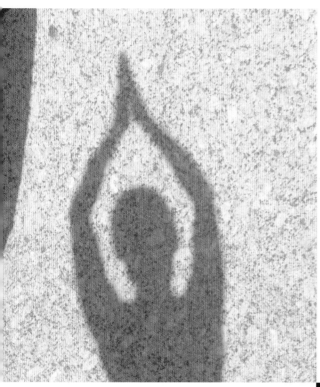

mines how you feel and extends to how you look. This offers a sustainable solution: the stronger your feeling of health and wellbeing, the stronger your self-esteem. This, in turn, makes you less likely to allow criticism (your own, or other people's) of your body, based on unrealistic ideals, to undermine your ability to focus on attaining good health.

In good health, your attractiveness and beauty shine through. And once you have achieved good health, you may discover that you are within a healthy weight range.

HEALTH FROM THE INSIDE OUT

Health is feeling great. It is an experience that can be felt from the inside out. It is the result of all body systems functioning optimally. It is also the result of

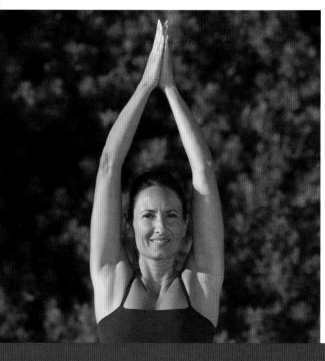

mental and emotional health—your attitude towards yourself and your life and your ability to navigate emotional ups and downs with skill and adaptability.

Your health, and how you feel in and about your body, changes constantly. Some days you feel great, others not. You should strive to feel healthy most of the time. You also need resilience—life is about finding and losing balance. Health is not a fixed state of being. It is a dynamic process involving the practice of returning to balance again and again.

Living in a state of balanced health most of the time requires stamina. Once you accept this, your journey into health is more likely to be sustainable.

Yoga postures, breathing and mindful awareness practices are training ground for optimal physical functioning and psychological health. Yoga has centuries behind it to prove its effectiveness in developing your fitness, a comfortable, confident posture, a sense of vitality, emotional resilience, mental clarity and fine-tuned awareness.

A LONG-TERM, SUSTAINABLE SOLUTION

This book is not a quick fix for losing large amounts of weight in a short time, without addressing the root cause of your weight problem. Quick fixes, like crash dieting, may lead to quick weight loss initially, but in the long run actually lead to weight gain. Not only do you regain the weight you lost, but you go beyond where you started in the first place. Your body responds to a crash diet by going into famine mode. This involves storing fat more readily than before as a slow-burning source of energy. This is a result of your metabolism slowing down in order to conserve the energy from the little food you are eating. When you start eating normally again, your body picks up weight quickly, continuing to store fat as if in famine mode. It is possible to reverse the detrimental effects of crash dieting, but it takes time, perseverance and dedication to health. And just in case you are thinking 'Well, just one more crash diet' remember that the longer you persist with unhealthy diet options, the harder it will be for you to move into health.

At times you may doubt or become impatient. At such times, simply consider the cost to your health and well-being of doing nothing or persisting with unsustainable, quick-fix weight-loss solutions.

SOME IDEA OF TIME

How unhealthily you have been eating, and for how long, together with how infrequently you have been exercising, will influence how quickly health and ideal weight are achieved.

When you start applying the tools of this book, there may be an initial period during which you experience detoxification symptoms or some physical discomfort, However, within a week or two you generally move through the worst of these symptoms and establish the beginnings of a familiar routine. It is said to take 21 days to break a habit, so this is another marker to look forward to as your new lifestyle habits become ingrained.

By then you will definitely notice some weight loss, with accompanying benefits, such as increased energy levels and a more positive outlook on life, as encouragement to continue. Following this is a three-month mark, by which time the routine is well established and there is an increased consistency in your experience of health.For different people it takes different lengths of time to achieve ideal weight and shape. Persevere. In time your efforts will pay off.

Know Thyself

This chapter is an opportunity to know yourself better through your physical body. This includes an introduction to three basic body types, and recommendations for exercise and lifestyle patterns that would be most beneficial for each body type.

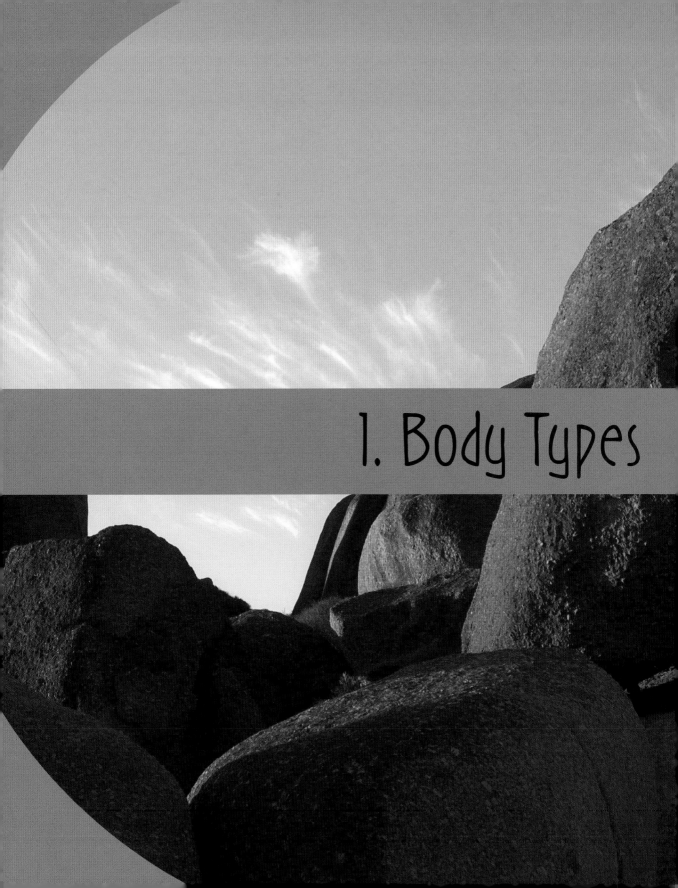

1. Body Types

In health, no body type is over or underweight

THREE BODY TYPES

There are three basic body types that are genetically determined. Although body type is a basic structure that cannot be changed, health and relative body weight can. The body types are described here in terms of leanness, muscularity and roundness of the body. They correspond with two well-known systems of body type classification, which are the Ayurvedic body types of Vata, Pitta and Kapha, and the Western system of Somatyping bodies as Ectomorph, Mesomorph and Endomorph.

This chapter is your invitation to accept your body type or genetic constitution. It is a starting point from which health and a realistic body image can develop.

COMBINATIONS

A person can be a combination of two or all three body types, although one type is usually dominant. Most people are a combination of two body types. A person might be a muscular-round body type—predominantly round, with tendency to store fat easily, as well as being strong and muscular. In that case muscle definition will be concealed by a slightly rounded appearance. In maturity lean persons may develop a tendency to accumulate fatty tissue, but their physique generally will remain more slender than a truly round body type.

The Western societal ideal is the lean body type, or a combination of muscular and lean, like an athlete. The female ideal in this culture is lean, and the male ideal is muscular. These ideals are very difficult, and often unhealthy, for a person with a round body type to achieve.

This chapter is an invitation to love and accept your body, knowing that radiant good health and beauty will transcend your body type. When this inner beauty shines through, it can surpass that of people with a supposedly ideal body shape, but who have not accessed their own inner shine, their glow of health. It is also an invitation to honour diversity, to celebrate your uniqueness and that of others. So why not permit yourself to live in the glow of your health and well-being?

LEAN BODY TYPE

[Equivalent: Vata; Ectomorph]

PHYSIQUE: Tendency to be slender, possibly with a fragile appearance. Lean, long muscles.

ENERGY LEVEL: Energy comes in bursts, followed by a period of low energy.

APPETITE: Can have a small appetite to feed their slight frame. Tendency to eat irregularly.

WEIGHT/SHAPE ISSUE: Have a fast metabolism leading to minimal fat being stored on the body. There may be a tendency to be underweight. This body type can also accumulate fatty deposits on the body, for instance, through nervous eating. Young people with this body type can lose weight quickly and easily when they set their minds to it. Achieving and maintaining muscular tone is generally the more challenging issue for this body type.

YOGA RECOMMENDATION: This body type calls for more gentle or low-impact exercise than the other body types, with the focus on body toning and strength-building to help support their fragile frame. This also helps prevent loose, sagging flesh with progressively bonier appearance later in life. The body toning sessions in chapter 6 are beneficial in support of this. Also all Vinyasa in chapter 7 can be beneficial.

A generally helpful factor for this body type is regularity: of eating, exercise, sleep and of lifestyle in general. This helps to develop a constant energy level.

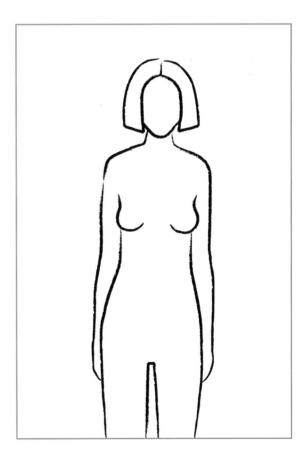

MUSCULAR BODY TYPE

[Equivalent: Pitta; Mesomorph]

PHYSIQUE: Muscular and often big-boned.

ENERGY LEVEL: Moderate energy level and endurance. Can come alive when challenged, rising to the task with higher energy output to see it through. Muscular tension can deplete energy.

APPETITE: Regular eating patterns, large appetite, strong digestion.

WEIGHT/SHAPE ISSUE: Tendency to have a fast metabolism and a strong digestive system. This body type can be thick with muscle, with very little fat. Women of this type might judge their physique as thicker and more solid than the ideals depicted by fashion models. This can lead to rejection of body shape. When over-eating as part of a self-destructive pattern, this body type can accumulate excess fat. They tend to lose weight fairly quickly, partly due to strong digestion, partly due to self-discipline if they set their minds to it.

YOGA RECOMMENDATION: It is important for persons of this body type to work on flexibility to balance strength and muscular build-up. This can improve general agility and ease in movement. People with this body type tend to enjoy working out and so might enjoy any of the sessions or posture sequences offered in this book. They often enjoy sport and Yoga can be used to complement the activity and help develop the body in a balanced, more comprehensive manner.

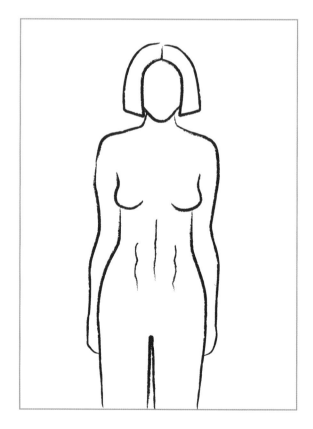

ROUND BODY TYPE

[Equivalent: Kapha and Endomorph]

PHYSIQUE: Tendency to be round and soft with smooth contours when healthy. Prone to excess fat accumulation and obesity when unhealthy.

ENERGY LEVEL: Steady energy with endurance. When out of balance, with excess weight accumulation, this type can feel heavy and sluggish, which will deplete energy. Their tendency is to sleep deeply and well and may struggle to wake up in the morning, appreciating a caffeine boost to kick-start their metabolism. This type benefits from exercising in the morning, possibly as caffeine substitute.

APPETITE: Because of fat reserves, the tendency is to feel only mild hunger. However, also tend to eat for emotional reasons, for self-nurturing, especially when feeling rejected by others or when comparing their bodies to that of the social ideal.

WEIGHT/SHAPE ISSUE: Tendency to have a slow metabolism and digestion. Weight loss can be slow. In modern times, this body type may be considered the least desirable. For that reason they may suffer from self-rejection and a dislike of their own bodies. In health, this body type is not overweight and can have a beautiful physical appearance, with attractive curves. Sensuality and grace of movement come more naturally to this body type than to others.

YOGA RECOMMENDATION: Regular routines should incorporate aerobic exercise to counter the tendency to sluggishness and to store excess fat. A regular Yoga practice, with an aerobic component, can increase energy levels.

Keeping the body flexible and strong also cultivates a feeling of relative lightness in this physique. It can also boost energy levels and general health by, for instance, improving digestion and cardiovascular health. The sessions outlined in chapter 6 are designed to achieve this balance. These sessions will also strengthen the body to develop a toned and agile physique. Even when toned and healthy, this body type generally has a somewhat rounded appearance.

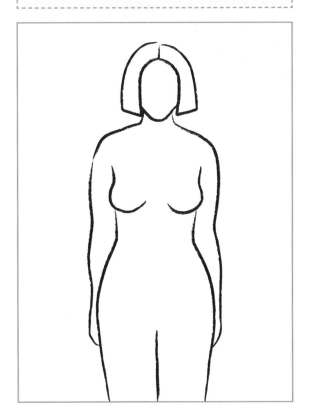

Fit and Fabulous

This chapter explains the role of fitness and body tone in achieving ideal weight and shape. It is not enough to change your diet. To achieve a shape in which you feel fabulous, you need physical fitness with accompanying body tone.

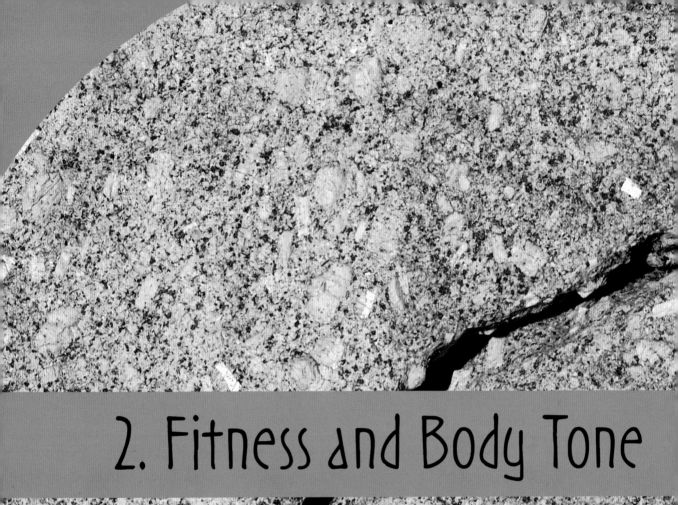

2. Fitness and Body Tone

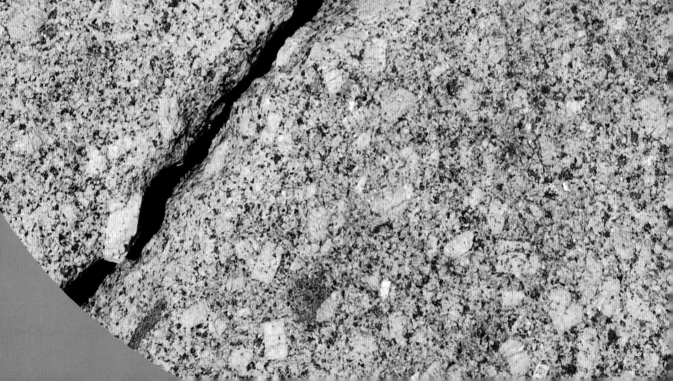

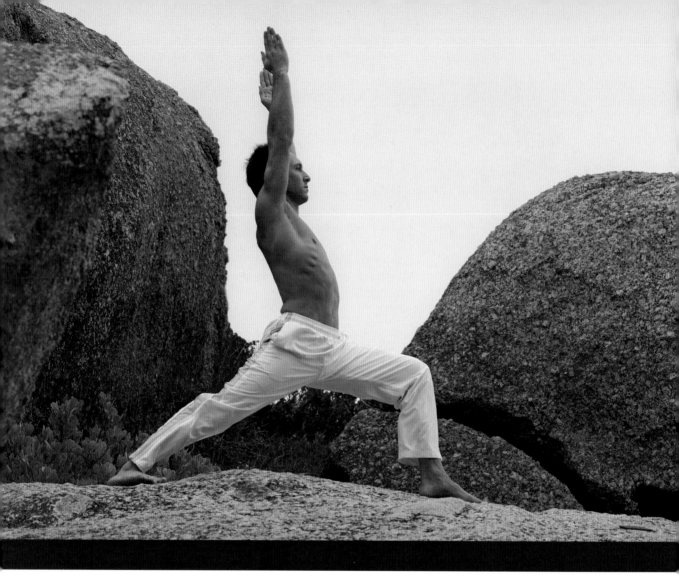

Defining Physical Fitness

Physical fitness can be defined as a state of physical readiness, resilience and relative agility, with a capacity for endurance. Health and fitness go hand in hand: overall health is an essential foundation of physical fitness; and fitness promotes overall health.

Cardiovascular fitness (and respiratory and circulatory health) supports the maintenance of a balanced, healthy metabolism for stable energy levels and weight regulation.

Physical fitness can help you get moving—literally and metaphorically. Physically it boosts your energy levels and metabolic rate, which helps you achieve your ideal weight. Metaphorically it gets you moving because feeling fit is inherently motivational.

In Hatha Yoga, physical fitness is the basis for achieving balanced, comfortable posture. This is conducive to sustained spiritual awareness. It is also helpful for sitting for long periods of time in meditation if one so desires.

Fitness is a function of three factors operating together. These factors support each other to achieve comfort, ease and poise in posture and movement.

In no particular order of importance, the three factors are:
» *Flexibility—for range of motion and the experience of 'openness', or lightness in one's physical experience.*
» *Strength—for stability and power in stillness and motion.*
» *Mobility—for agility, ease and endurance in motion.*

BODY TONE

Body tone serves by sculpting your body into fine form. Muscle tone helps improve circulation in those areas that may have excess fatty deposits. It also firms up areas of low muscle tone. Body tone is not only aesthetically appealing, it also promotes health by ensuring good posture, which supports the positioning, and therefore efficient function, of internal organs.

POSTURE

Balanced posture is centred between the opposing forces of grounding and uplift. Healthy posture can help prevent excess fat accumulation by avoiding postural imbalance or sagging, which can compress certain body areas, making them prone to fatty deposit accumulation.

There is also a link between posture and self-confidence, which plays a role in achieving and maintaining your ideal weight and shape.

TONING INSIDE AND OUT

Yoga is a system designed to tone the body inside and out. On the inside, Yoga postures massage and tone the internal organs, improving blood and lymph circulation and generally supporting healthy body system functioning. This is achieved through postures and posture combinations where opposing body parts are set up to stretch, compress or twist each other in support of healthy functioning. This improves circulation to and from all body tissues.

Breathing practices in Yoga promote health by enhancing lung capacity while oxygenating and energising all body systems and promoting healthy circulation.

Yoga postures balance strength building and flexibility training. This physical agility is discernible on the outside as fine posture and body tone relative to your body type.

FITNESS FOR LIFE

The kind of physical fitness promoted through Yoga is not seen as preparation for improved performance on any particular playing field. The playing field is life in general.

Hatha Yoga is seen as an exercise system for improving your performance when walking, moving and functioning in life. Yoga practice, maintained on a regular basis, can improve your energy levels, endurance and sense of being physically comfortable in your body. It also fine-tunes posture and movement to achieve optimal health and to enrich your experience of being alive.

PHYSICAL ENDURANCE AND YOGA

Physical endurance requires a strong heart muscle, as well as strong skeletal muscles.

Hatha Yoga is designed to improve physical endurance through the holding of postures. Breathing practice increases lung capacity and promotes oxygenation of body and brain tissues. The combination of postures and breathing improves blood and lymph circulation throughout the body. You will notice over time, with the regular practice of Yoga, that your capacity for aerobic exercise increases, as will your performance in any physically challenging activity or sport.

There is another factor that affects physical

endurance: your thoughts and the way you react to them, can deplete your energy reserves and thus reduce physical endurance.

In this regard Yoga can help by increasing awareness and promoting mental– emotional resilience, clarity and calm. This is achieved through the practice of postures, executed with breath awareness, and meditation.

THE HEART MUSCLE AND AEROBIC EXERCISE

In order to keep the heart muscle strong, aerobic exercise is required. Aerobic means 'with air' or oxygen. The American College of Sports Medicine (ACSM) defines aerobic exercise as 'any activity that uses large muscle groups, can be maintained continuously, and is rhythmic in nature.' It is a type of exercise that overloads the heart and lungs and causes them to work harder than at rest. Aerobic exercise promotes fat-burning and weight loss. It increases oxygen supply to the muscles, the brain and all body tissues.

AN AEROBIC FORMULA

The generally agreed upon formula for aerobic exercise is to increase your heart rate to double its normal rate and to maintain this increased rate for at least 20 minutes at a time. To allow for this, extra time needs to be set aside to gradually increase the heart rate to a point where exercise becomes aerobic and, afterwards, to allow time for cooling down:

» Warm-up: a period of about 10 minutes is recommended to gradually warm up your muscles and raise your heart rate to the level where exercise becomes aerobic. One option is to carry out a few repetitions of one or more of the sequences offered in chapter 7. If you are walking, running, or doing

sport, you can also simply take an extra 10 minutes to start slowly, gradually building up to a pace you can maintain for 20 minutes.

» Maintaining your increased heart rate: Yoga can be used as an aerobic work-out. This can be achieved by carrying out many repetitions of sequences, such as the Sun Salutation versions offered in chapter 8, repeated for 20 minutes continuously. Another option is to walk, jog, or perform any other aerobic activity two or three days a week, alongside your practice of Yoga.

» Finally allow 5 or 10 minutes afterwards for cooling down to return to a rested state. There is a Yoga stretch and cool-down session offered in chapter 7 that you can use if you choose an aerobic activity other than Yoga.

There are programme ideas in chapter 6 to help you design your exercise week to include an aerobic component in conjunction with the Yoga sessions offered in this book.

MODERATE EXERTION

It is possible to overdo exercise. If you feel exhausted for a number of hours after exercising, you may be overdoing it. Aerobic exercise should not exceed the point where you can maintain a conversation. You should be breathing more deeply, or harder, than usual during aerobic exercise, with a steady rhythm to your breathing and without gasping for breath.

For effective fat burning, maximum exertion for short bursts of time is not as effective as moderate exertion for longer.

Exercise should be something you enjoy, so that you would want to do it again. In time, you may even come to crave exercise.

In order to keep the heart muscle strong, aerobic exercise is required.

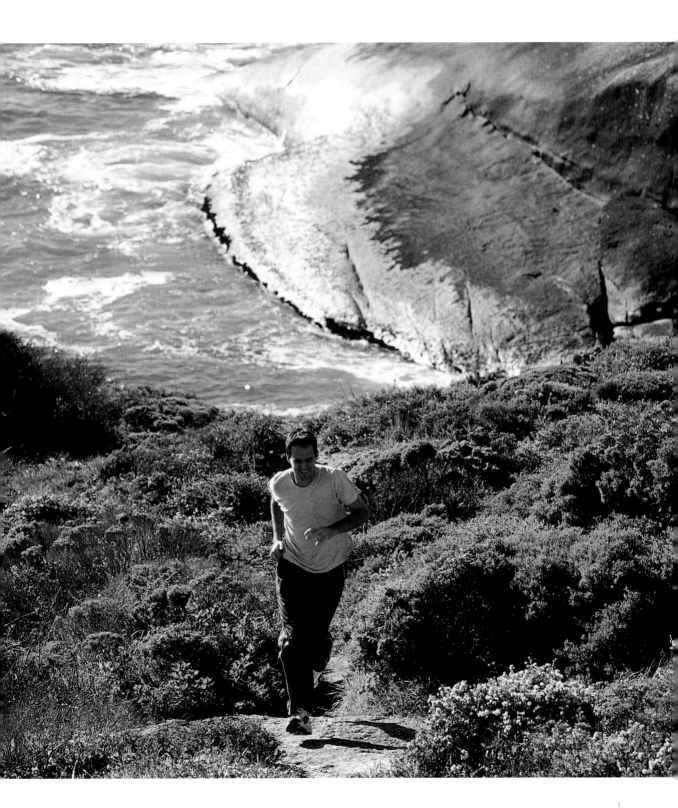

An all-round work-out

To achieve your ideal shape

For a programme to achieve and maintain ideal weight and shape, two basic components need to be included. There needs to be an aerobic component promoting fitness of the heart muscle and healthy metabolic rate. You also need exercise designed to promote overall body tone. This involves building strength and increasing flexibility in a balanced way, involving all body parts, and improving posture.

Running, walking and many sporting activities work certain body parts more than others and can, over time, lead to imbalance, and limit range of motion of certain joints. This can detract from healthy posture and reduce the feeling of well-being, energy levels, and health.

Yoga is one of the few systems that offers such an all round work-out. It can be used alone, or in conjunction with other activities; for improved performance at the sport of your choice; for general improvement in health; and for achieving and maintaining a balanced, comfortable posture. Yoga also reduces your risk of injury due to incorrect posture, movement or use of the body—whether in sport or daily activities.

Physical fitness and healthy bones

Bones are alive and, like muscles, require regular weight-bearing exercise to remain healthy and strong. The force of gravity helps to maintain bone density and health. The kind of exercise required should involve the pull of working muscles on bones in a variety of ways, for brief periods of time. Yoga is designed to address this, helping increase bone density, supporting healthy bones and skeletal structure.

Yoga also allows for posture and movement to place the least amount of stress and strain on the bones of the body. In this way, the skeleton is free to carry out its function optimally, of forming and maintaining the basic structure of the body.

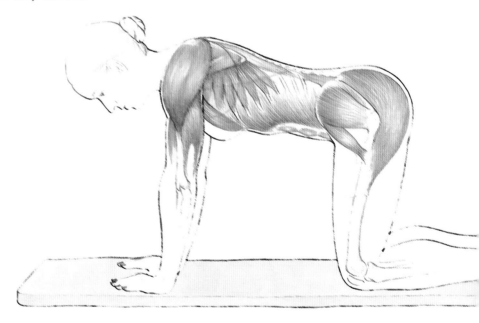

FITNESS AND METABOLISM

Metabolism is a function of the endocrine system, mainly regulated by the thyroid gland, which is located in the neck. The metabolic rate is the rate at which chemical reactions occur in every cell of the body, converting food and oxygen into energy. Metabolism also plays a role in determining whether food is converted into energy or stored as fat. In a balanced system, metabolism maintains an energy-efficient body.

Regular exercise and a healthy eating pattern promote metabolic health. Metabolism is also affected by emotions: speeding up or slowing down depending on how we feel.

HOW YOGA PROMOTES A HEALTHY METABOLISM

» Yoga can help speed up a slow metabolism, or help to calm and slow down a fast metabolism.
» Any Yoga posture that involves the neck, such as neck rolls and the shoulder stand, will tone the thyroid gland. All sessions in chapter 6 and the sequences in chapter 7 include components that tone the thyroid gland.
» Physical fitness, in general, however achieved, will promote metabolic health.
» Meditation and consistent Yoga posture practice can assist with mastery over the mind and emotions that influence metabolic rate.

HOW YOGA CAN HELP REDUCE

FAT DEPOSITS

» The sessions in chapter 6 are designed for slimming and toning of specific areas of the body and of the thyroid gland that regulates metabolism. Postures and posture combinations are designed to break down layers of excess fat deposits by squeezing, stretching and twisting the body. At the same time postures improve circulation to and from fatty tissue. The Yoga sessions in this book can also be used by slim people for general toning, health and weight maintenance.
» Cardiovascular exercise aids a healthy metabolism, which assists in fat loss. Multiple, continuous repetitions of the sequences in chapter 7 will serve the

Physical fitness promotes metabolic health

purpose. Or you can do aerobic exercise such as walking, running and swimming, in addition to Yoga.
» The fire breath, as used in the session for slimming and toning the waistline, has the effect of speeding up metabolism, increasing the rate at which fat is broken down in the body. It also can lead to improved circulation in general and improved skin tone.

CELLULITE

» 'Cellulite' is a term used to describe excess fatty deposits on the body. Cellulite is not a medical term. It is a term coined in European salons and spas. Medical authorities have found that cellulite is simply ordinary fatty tissue. Strands of fibrous tissue connect the skin to deeper tissue layers and also separate compartments that contain fat cells. When fat cells increase in size as excess fat accumulates, these compartments bulge and produce a waffled appearance of the skin.

» You can lose excess fat by intervening with a healthy diet, an exercise programme and other supportive tools such as body brushing and massage. These naturally lead you in the direction of health with accompanying loss of fat over time. With patience and persistence, you can achieve a body in which only a healthy amount of fat exists.

CAUSES OF EXCESS FAT

» Poor nutrition from eating foods that are not conducive to health, and often in excess.
» Repeated crash dieting.
» Sedentary lifestyle with insufficient or perhaps complete lack of exercise
» A hormonal imbalance as a result of the first two factors of poor nutrition and a sedentary lifestyle. Hormonal imbalance can also be due to medication, psychological factors, pregnancy or some form of ill-health of the endocrine or other body system. In such cases a weight loss program may need to be carried out in conjunction with appropriate medical or other specialist attention.

Various factors helping to reduce fatty deposits are exercise, regular massage and body brushing.

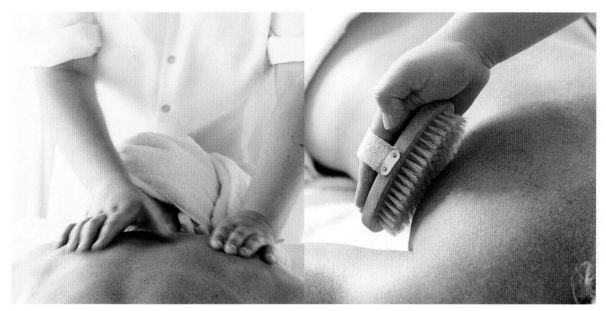

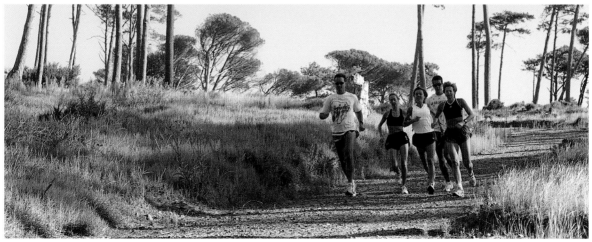

What Yoga Can Offer

Psychological factors often contribute to being over or underweight. Out of habit, and because it is so abundantly availabile, people start reaching for food to fill needs other than hunger. Some people use food deprivation as a way to feel in control of their lives. Either way, food is used to induce calm and content-ment when stressed or lonely, and this can become confused with feelings of true hunger. In this way it is possible to lose touch with your natural rhythms and authentic needs.

In the moment, food may feel nur-turing and fulfilling. However, in the long run, these habits will lead you further into misery rather than health.

Most people know what is healthy, yet do not live accordingly. The reason for this is psychological. Your attitude towards your health determines what you do about it.

Whether or not you choose health in each moment is primarily influenced by the way you manage your emotional life and stress.

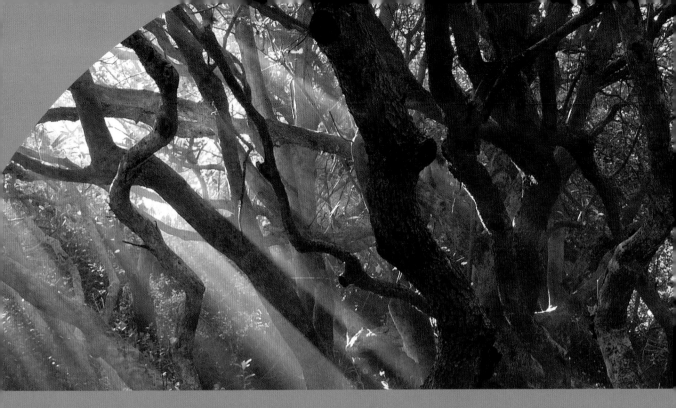
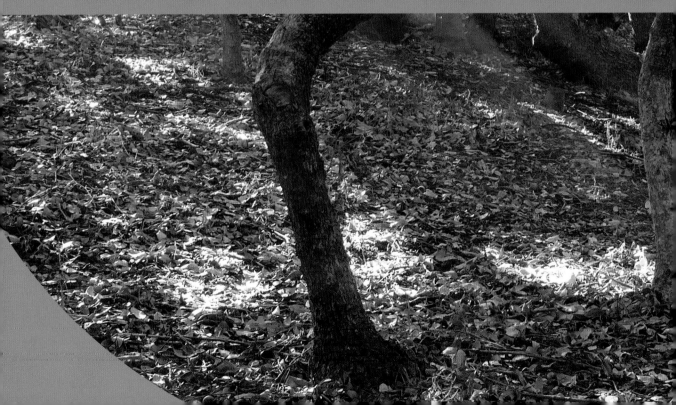

3. Psychology of Weight Loss

» *Emotional insecurity, often due to feeling unful-filled, unaccepted or challenged.*

» *Fat can seem a protective buffer between you and the world.*

» *A need to nurture or be nurtured.*

» *Food can help you feel more grounded and calm.*

» *In some cultures obesity is a sign of wealth and beauty.*

Yoga and Psychology

According to the Kosha system in Yogic philosophy, the nature of being human encompasses physical and psychological aspects that function as one holistic system. The Kosha system refers to these different aspects as layers of subjective experience. Layers range from the dense physical body to the more subtle levels of emotions, mind and spirit. Psychology refers to the emotional, mental and spiritual aspects of our being. Together, all aspects make up our subjective experience of being alive.

Layers influence each other. For example, our thoughts and emotions influence physical posture and breathing patterns; while our posture and breathing influence our thoughts and feelings. Posture is a reflection of our psychological attitude towards our lives and our selves. It also offers a tangible way of meeting our psychological needs through their expression in physical form.

Thought patterns and emotions can result in a body posture and breathing patterns that can become fixed over time. This results in a situation where the body, in turn, then perpetuates thought patterns and emotions.

Unhealthy posture results from high levels of muscle tension or collapse that can be detrimental to body and mind. A fit and toned body with balanced, comfortable posture is not only healthy, it also breaks the physical link to harmful ways of thinking and feeling.

Although you may not always be aware of your posture, or moment-to-moment postural shifts, you can train yourself to become more aware and influential.

Yoga offers practical tools for achieving a posture that is comfortable, supportive and empowering. The knowledge that it is possible to influence your shape in this way in itself can be empowering. It cultivates a sense of confidence in your ability to navigate life's ups and downs more skillfully.

Yoga for psychological health

» The physical and mental centring attained through Yoga postures and meditation can help cultivate a deep, sustainable inner peacefulness. This can help you remain centred in the face of emotional storms and help control cravings and addictive behaviour. It also helps you think more clearly more consistently.

» Yoga also promotes breath awareness, through attention to breath in postures and meditation. This

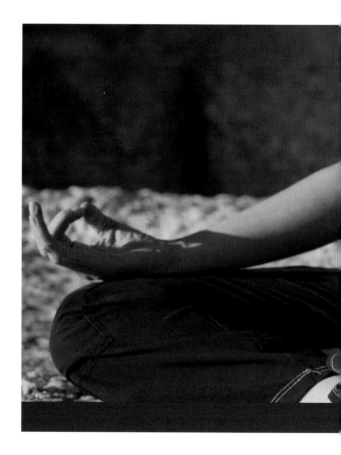

enables you to maintain calm, steady breathing. Breath and emotions are intimately connected. Breathing is influenced by emotions. When a strong emotion is present, for instance, breathing gets shallow, or irregular, restricted or fast. Conversely, by controlling your breathing, you can improve your sense of well-being by controlling your reactions in an emotional situation.

» Breathing that is calm, full and steady goes with clearer thinking and with a mental–emotional state that is calm and steady.

» Together, the basic elements in Hatha Yoga practice —posture, breathing and mental focus—cultivate a state of balance in body and mind.

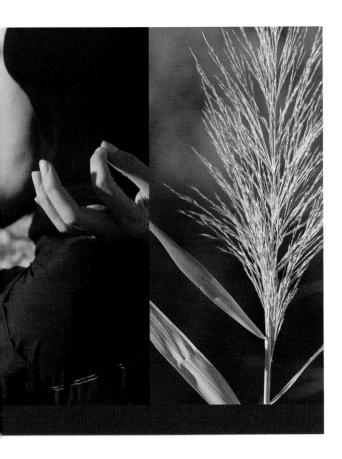

WHAT LIGHTS YOU UP?

When you're in love, or feeling inspired, it affects you physically and psychologically. The nervous and endocrine systems generate a delightful, perhaps blissful, quality felt as warmth and lightness in your physical body.

This state of feeling 'aglow' with inspiration or love is conducive to good health, feeding the cells of your body with vitality. This can have a motivating effect, awakening your desire to be creative in line with your passions and inspirations. It also tends to awaken a more caring attitude toward yourself and others.

If you do not allow for an outlet for that which inspires you, the sense of frustration can deplete your energy. Perhaps it comes along with feeling that life is meaningless to you and that you have no contribution to make.

Everyone has something to contribute, something that can help you feel your life is meaningful. This can give you a reason to get out of bed in the morning, so as to take even one tiny step toward your goals.

Identifying an inspiring vision for your future, with practical, achievable goals worth living for, also extends your attention beyond a potentially obsessive focus on your body alone. It helps you focus on that into which you want to channel your new-found energy and vitality.

Ideal weight and shape are not final goals. Rather, they are keys to unlocking your vitality for living a more fulfilling, rewarding, energised life toward dreams that inspire you.

In Yoga, love and inspiration are gateways to health, spiritual awareness and evolution. The longer we can bask in the glow of our love and inspiration, and function from this place in the context of practical, material reality, the more consistent our experience of physical and psychological well-being. This may mean being kind to yourself and others in times of challenge. It can also be helpful to identify a spiritual purpose for you in a challenging situation.

At times, when your life is on an even keel, you may want to invite the feeling of love to fill you just for the sake of it; or to tune in to an inspiring thought; or to create inspiring goals and start planning your way towards them.

A Yoga practice can serve as a means of cultivating a simple love of life through investing time in your well-being. Yoga practices also open your body, clear your mind and offer you a way to tune in to your spirit each day. Yoga is your means of plugging into living a switched-on life of radiant vitality.

Practised on the Yoga mat and applied in life, the skills taught in Yoga can offer perspective and generally strengthen your resolve to meet obstacles that threaten to sabotage your progress as life unfolds. Your new skills develop your capacity to function responsibly and serve your best interests in the long run. This in turn promotes love of life, as you achieve good results and gain confidence in your abilities.

ADDICTIONS, CRAVINGS AND SELF-DESTRUCTIVE BEHAVIOUR—UNHEALTHY STRESS MANAGEMENT

Most people know what it takes to be healthy. It appears logical to choose health and vitality over ill-health and physical depletion. However, many people do not choose health all the time, instead choosing to sabotage their health, doing what they know is not good for them.

Whether or not you choose health in each moment is influenced by the way you manage your emotions and stress.

The root of unhealthy addictions is giving in to cravings without thinking rationally about what it is you really need at the time.

Over time your cravings begin to take charge of your behaviour and destroy your ability to think clearly enough to make conscious choices about your health. The behaviour becomes automatic and you may feel you no longer have a choice, feeling stuck in a habit of acting before thinking.

THE CHALLENGE

The challenge is to develop an inner witness to your experience. The function of this inner witness is to monitor impulsive, perhaps habitual, emotional responses played out with food or other addictive substance or activity, replacing it with conscious choice, preferably in line with health of mind and body in the long run.

Over time, unhealthy patterns will lose their power over you. As you move into health, you actually begin to crave healthy foods and activities.

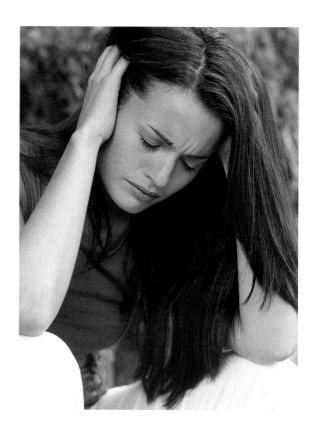

We cannot make emotions and life challenges go away. What we can do is transform our reactions to them.

TIPS TO HELP YOU MEET THIS CHALLENGE

» *Pause for a moment before you act or eat. This is a tool to help impulse control, inviting the rational brain to have its say. It creates a time gap between the impulse and the action; a time for changing the course of behavior in service of well-being in the long run.*

» *Supportive touch can be helpful. It serves as a first aid to help you make best use of a pausing moment. It can help you to literally get in touch with yourself when feeling emotionally or mentally challenged. It helps quiet the mind and soothe emotional turbulence, gradually taming insistent cravings. While taking a few deep breaths, you can place your hands over you heart; hold your hands together in the prayer pose; hold your head with one hand behind and one hand either on top of or in front of your head. You can also try a Yoga technique called Yoni or Sanmukhi Mudra: place the fingers of both hands over your closed eyes, ears, nose (only partially blocking air passage so you can still breathe through your nose) and lips, as if to seal these 'sense doors.'*

» *Think about what you really need. For example, if you want food, ask yourself if you are really hungry for food or for emotional comfort. Perhaps you need a channel for your emotions and the energy generated by them. Perhaps you need to say something to someone.*

» *Consider the possibility that you may fear your own success. People sometimes fear success more than failure, which may be more familiar, and seem comfortable and less threatening. Let your health and aspirations take control. With practice you can train yourself to maintain this focus.*

Touch, even for a few quiet breaths, has a soothing effect that can help you think more clearly.

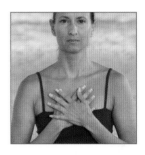

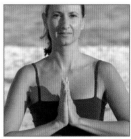

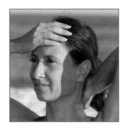
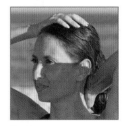

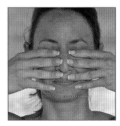

Vibrant Health

Achieving and maintaining vibrant health requires attention to diet, exercise and other lifestyle factors. Ideal weight and shape are natural products of this vibrant health. Doing physical exercise, without attention to diet and other lifestyle factors, makes the exercise far less effective. Poor nutrition, lack of sleep or lack of fresh air will, at best, hinder your progress and your enjoyment of your physical Yoga practice. At worst it can render your efforts ineffective.

This chapter makes recommendations about diet and other lifestyle factors. Some are crucial to a health-oriented weight-loss programme, others are offered as supportive ideas.

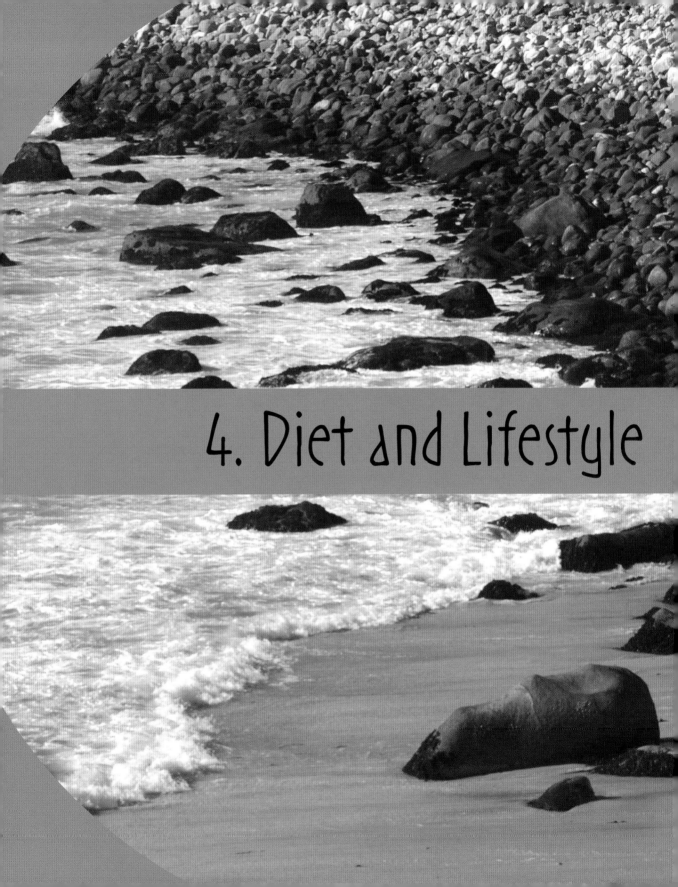

4. Diet and Lifestyle

Diet

Diet plays a central role in weight loss. Strict, calorie-counting diets, or crash diets, lead to swift weight loss initially, which is rapidly regained—and then some—as soon as normal eating is resumed. The focus should be on establishing healthy and sustainable eating patterns.

A Yogic perspective

According to Yogic philosophy, foods influence psychological as well as physical health. According to the Yogic system there are three general categories, called *Guna,* relating to human psychology, and reflected in the body. They are *Sattva*, associated with balance and purity; *Rajas,* associated with agitation, passion and aggression; and *Tamas* associated with inertia and depression.

Guna is a Sanskrit word that means a quality or constituent of nature. The different *Guna* influence and are influenced by physical and psychological factors, food being one factor. Certain foods are conducive to certain qualities.

Tamasic: When overweight, there is usually a Tamasic tendency in the diet. A Tamasic diet is energy depleting and lacks nutrition. It includes foods that are not fresh, may be highly processed, and heavy or oily. Eating heavy foods such as red meat on a regular basis is Tamas producing. Alcohol, in the long run, also leads to a Tamasic state.

Rajasic: Rajasic foods have a stimulating, heating effect on the body. They can promote fat-burning, but in excess can lead to digestive discomfort, ill-health and mental agitation. Examples are: spicy foods; refined sugar; and any extreme flavour, such as very bitter, salty or pungent. Onions and garlic are also considered Rajasic. A general recommendation is not to over-spice food. The less you flavour food, the more you get used to appreciating natural flavours. Your ability to appreciate natural flavours diminishes when you too often eat food that is highly salted or spiced. Salt also causes water retention, so use it sparingly.

When consumed in excess, Rajasic foods can disturb the inner sense of quiet, peace and contentment.

Physical exercise has a Rajasic effect on the body and, when not overdone, exercise can help the body make the transition from a Tamasic to a Sattvic state.

Sattvic: A Sattvic diet promotes health and energy; mental clarity and a calm state of being conducive to emotional health. It is also associated with the Yogic aspiration of an internal awakened state of consciousness. A Sattvic diet is rich in fresh, natural foods and creates a slightly alkaline environment for optimal digestion and health.

Alkaline diet and digestion

A diet should create a slightly alkaline environment in the digestive system and blood. This requires food to be combined in particular ways.

Note: In Yogic literature, a vegetarian diet is not considered essential, though recommended for more advanced practitioners to attain awareness of progressively subtler aspects of the human experience, associated with spirituality. Following is an indication of how to include meat, fish and eggs in your diet in a way that creates an alkaline environment in your system. If you are eating meat, fish and eggs, opt for the meat of animals allowed relative freedom over those kept in highly restricted living conditions. Also inquire as to whether the animals are fed hormones or some form of growth supplement. Avoid ones that are.

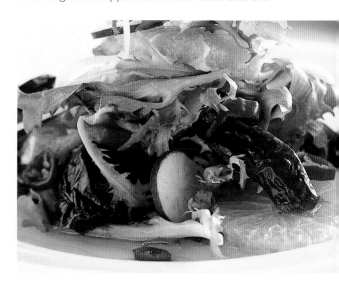

BASIC RECOMMENDATIONS FOR A NATURAL,
HEALTH-PROMOTING DIET:

» *Eat foods as close to their natural, fresh state as possible: fresh fruit, vegetables, grains and pulses rather than canned, frozen or highly processed foods.*

» *Eat until you are satisfied, not till you feel full. This helps digestion as well as agility, mental clarity and beautiful appearance.*

» *Eat slowly and chew your food well.*

» *Eat three times a day: two light and one heavy meal. In hot months, one of these can be fruit only. A general rule is to wait at least three or four hours between meals. If you eat fruit, wait an hour or two before eating more fruit or moving on to other kinds of foods.*

» *Break the habit of snacking between meals. If you are really hungry, snack on fresh or dried fruit and nuts for a quick energy boost to see you through to mealtime. Drinking water can help you feel satisfied between meals.*

» *Eat your largest meal at midday. If this does not fit into a working and family schedule, try to eat your large meal as early as possible in the evening, allowing at least two hours before going to sleep.*

» *Keep caffeine to a minimum. In small amounts it can have an uplifting, stimulating effect, though too much caffeine taxes your adrenal glands and affects your immune system, weight regulation and emotional stability.*

» *Avoid alcohol, smoking and other intoxicants, since these interfere with healthy body system functioning and mental health.*

» *Replace refined sugar with honey, fructose or dried fruits.*

» *Get in the habit of checking ingredients on food packaging, and avoid foods with preservatives, colourants, artificial sweeteners and other additives.*

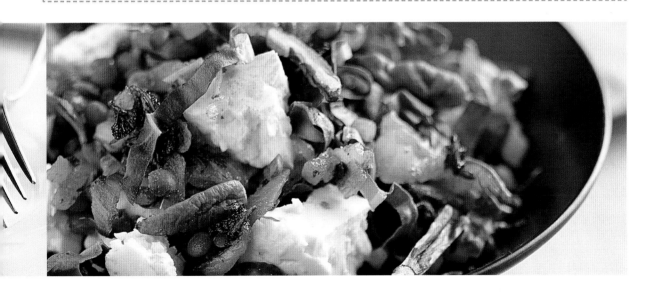

BASIC GUIDELINES FOR AN ALKALINE DIET

» *Eat carbohydrates and concentrated proteins at separate meals. Vegetables, apart from potato, which is carbohydrate, can be combined with either carbohydrates or proteins. For example, you can eat carbohydrates such as rice, bread, potatoes, pasta or any grain with vegetables and salads at one meal. If you are eating concentrated protein, such as meat, fish, eggs, soya or tofu, nuts and dairy products, combine it with vegetables and salads, rather than with carbohydrates. Legumes, such as peas, lentils and mung beans, should be combined with a grain such as rice. Legumes and grains are not complete proteins but complement each other and need to be eaten together so that you can get the complete protein. This combination should not disturb your digestion.*

» *Eat fruit on its own, or combined with other fruits, nuts or seeds, and preferably on an empty stomach. This is because fruit tends to ferment in the digestive tract when it cannot pass through your system fairly quickly. This can compromise digestion.*

» *Drinking directly after a meal interferes with digestion. It is said to pour water over the fire of digestion. Drink before a meal or between meals. If you do wish to have some liquid after a meal, wait at least half an hour before drinking a small amount of liquid.*

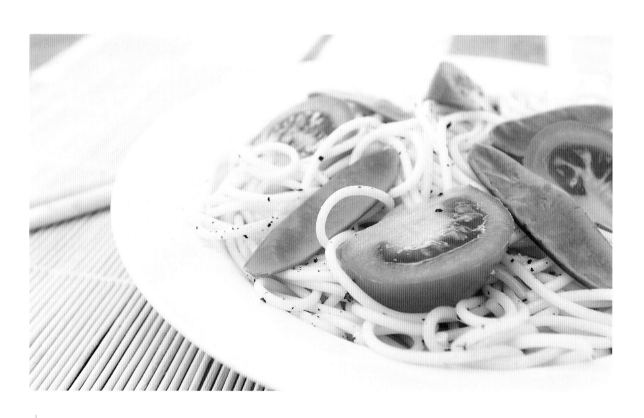

GOOD FAT, BAD FAT

Essential fatty acids are called essential because that is what they are to your health. Each cell in your body and all body systems need a certain amount of fat to function. Fat serves as an insulator, and plays an important role in immune system functioning as well as reproductive health. It is also a slow-burning energy reserve for times of need.

It is recommended to keep your unsaturated fat intake moderate to small. However, you definitely need to include it in your daily diet. Examples of sources of unsaturated fats are avocados, bananas, nuts, seeds and cold-pressed oils, such as olive oil or flax (linseed) oil.

Saturated fat is not generally conducive to health. (Coconut is an exception.) In the modern diet saturated fats are usually consumed in fast foods, especially when fried, or the fat on red meat.

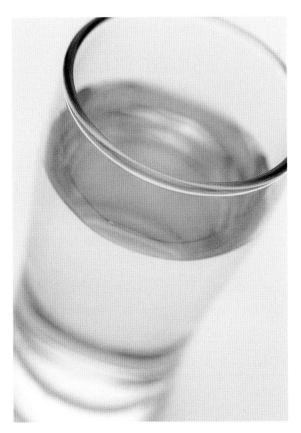

When using oil with cooked food, it is recommended to add oils at the end of the cooking process so that the oil does not get heated to boiling or sizzling temperature. It is possible to stir-fry vegetables in water, adding water gradually as needed, then adding cold-pressed oil, such as olive or sesame oil at the end of the process. If you wish to use some oil for stir-frying, grapeseed oil is considered one of the most heat-resistant oils for frying purposes.

WATER FOR WEIGHT LOSS AND HEALTH

Water plays an essential part in the healthy functioning of all body systems. It literally has the effect of flushing your system clean.

It is recommended to drink between six and eight glasses of water a day, preferably at room temperature. Drinking a few cups of hot water each day may help weight loss.

It is possible to overdo water consumption to the detriment of healthy body system functioning. A way to monitor this is to avoid forcing water down your throat when you really do not want it or have simply had enough for the time being. Thirst can also at times be mistaken for hunger so, as a general rule, get in the habit of drinking some water before food when you feel like eating.

Healthy diet most of the time

Know from the start that there will be times when you deviate from healthy eating. This is natural. It is, however, important to keep these times in check lest they begin to take charge of your eating patterns, overriding your inner knowledge of what is supportive of your health and ideal weight in the long run.

Remember: health that is sustainable means a constant state of moving out of and returning into balance. Whenever you deviate from health, consider it as an opportunity to challenge your inner strength to steer you back into health.

OTHER ESSENTIAL LIFESTYLE FACTORS

» *Balance of work, rest and play: each is important, though not necessarily in the same proportion. For example, if you work many hours a day and week, be sure to allow some rest time at the end of each working day. Schedule one day off work each week for leisure or play; spend extra time in nature, or make time for a hobby. Also make time for a holiday each year—an extended period of rest and rejuvenation.*

» *Sufficient sleep and rest: if you struggle to relax at night, try doing one of the calming, soothing Yoga sequences a few times before going to bed to help unwind and promote restfulness. While lying in bed, for relaxation, you can also try the holds described on p. 37— touching your head or your heart, or the mudra with fingers over your eyes, ears, nose and mouth. Hold them for as long as you feel you need, while breathing naturally.*

» *Spend time outdoors breathing fresh air and absorbing sunshine or natural daylight even if the sun is not shining. This supports health in body and mind. At least 20 minutes a day outdoors is recommended. You can build this into your daily routine, perhaps going for a walk outdoors daily or eating your lunch outdoors.*

» *Hygiene, including personal hygiene and keeping your environment clean, is important for your state of mind as well as physical health.*

» *Other lifestyle factors in Yogic philosophy pertain to a life of morality and right action. This includes ethical principles: non-violence, truthfulness and honesty as well as not falling prey to excess in any area of life.*

ADDITIONAL IDEAS TO HELP SLIMMING AND BODY TONING

» *Body brushing with a natural bristle brush or a loofah to improve circulation, especially over areas with an accumulation of excess fatty deposits. Always brush towards your heart or lymph nodes in the groin, armpits and neck.*

» *Regular massage for lymph drainage and improved circulation to and from areas of excess fatty deposit. You can hire a massage therapist for this; and you can massage areas of your own body, such as your legs, in the bath. This offers psychological nurturing.*

» *Living a meaningful life and setting goals is good for your health and state of mind. Having a sense of purpose in life, with practices to support it, offers a constructive avenue to channel your increased energy levels for the good of yourself, and perhaps others too. This encourages you to move beyond obsessive focus on the body; raising your head to look out in front of you to identify the contribution you can make; and what you can accomplish in your life. In so doing, body weight and shape are placed in healthy perspective in relation to the rest of your life.*

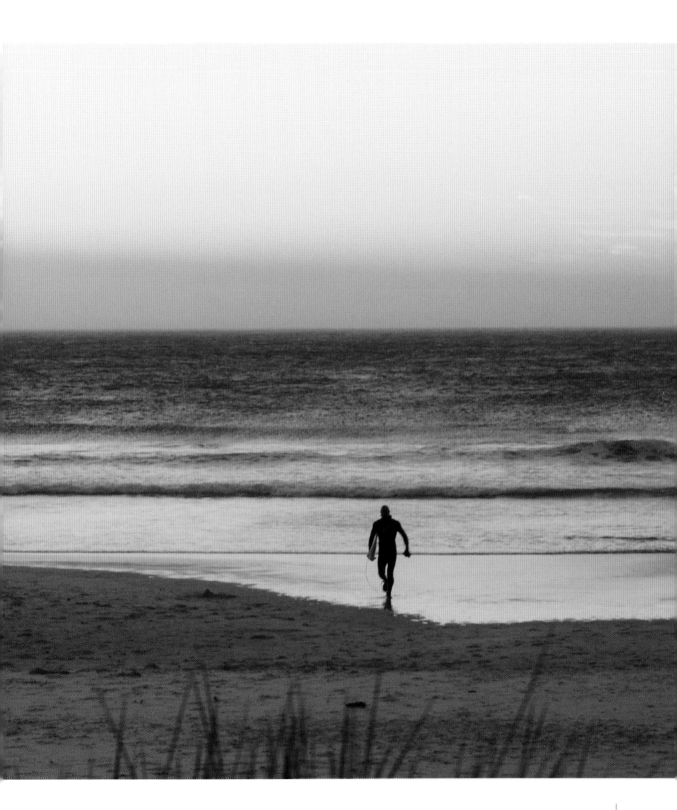

Before You Start

Read these instructions carefully before
you start moving into postures. The
instructions give recommended timing
for holding postures. The session plans
in chapter 6 include specific instructions
to invite grace, ease, lightness and
enjoyment into your postures.

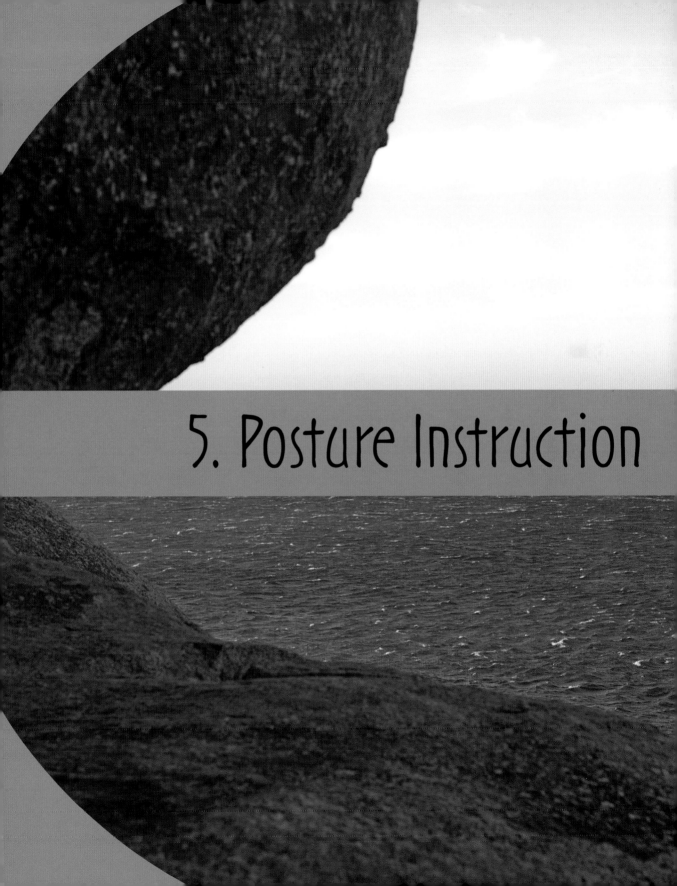

5. Posture Instruction

MEDITATION

STARTING POSITION: Sit in a comfortable cross-legged position, perhaps on a cushion. Or fold legs under so sitting on your heels in Vajrasana position with hands on thighs. (Avoid Vajrasana position if you have varicose veins.) Meditation can also be done sitting on a chair, preferably sitting upright rather than leaning into backrest. Eyes closed. Alternatively you can meditate with eyes open with steady focus on a point on the ground in front of you.

INSTRUCTION: Observe your natural breathing for a few minutes, focusing on breath at the entrance to your nostrils and on your upper lip area just below the nostrils, feeling the natural breath passing over this area. Ideally, allow 3 to 10 minutes at the end of a Yoga session. If meditating at a separate time of day, start with 5 minutes and work up to 20 minutes or more.

Meditation allows your mind to become sharper, clearer and more focused. It tames the mind's tendency to wander, while grounding and steadying your body and emotions. This can be very helpful to cultivate your will power and strengthen your resolve on your journey of achieving and maintaining ideal weight and shape.

PRANAYAMA
Breathing Practices

GENERAL NOTES:
» Eyes are closed for Pranayama unless otherwise specified.
» Breathing is through the nose unless otherwise specified.
» Sitting position for Pranayama, unless otherwise specified: Sit in a comfortable position, cross-legged, perhaps on a cushion or sit on your heels with legs folded under and hands on thighs. Or you can sit on a chair.

UJJAYI—Throat Breath

INSTRUCTION: With mouth closed, narrow the back of your throat, so that the flow of air on inhalation and exhalation passes through a narrower passage, making an extended 'hhhhh' sound from the back of your throat, a sound of sleep. This technique invites attention inwards, quietening the mind and replenishing the energy of the body as if asleep.

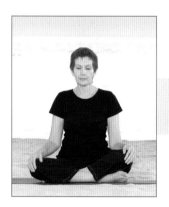
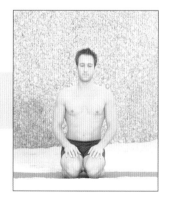

NADHI SODHANA
Alternate Nostril Breaths

The following technique is considered a simple preparatory exercise for the more advanced breathing technique of Nadhi Sodhana. For the purpose of this book, this technique is effective in developing balance between the right and left hemispheres of the brain and body correspondingly, and has a calming effect on the nerves.

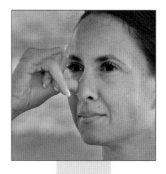

INSTRUCTION: Raise your right hand to place fourth (ring) finger and thumb on either side of your nostrils just below the bone so that with each finger alternately you can close off the air passage through one side of the nostril at a time. Curl your index and middle finger into your palm. Breathe deeply and evenly on inhalation and exhalation.

Start by closing off your left nostril with right fourth finger and exhaling through your right nostril, then inhale through the right nostril.

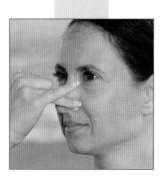

Then close right nostril with right thumb and exhale through your left nostril, followed by inhaling through your left nostril.

This completes one round. Repeat 8 rounds or more.

OPTION WITH PAUSES BETWEEN BREATHS: When you are well experienced in this breathing practice, you can practise pausing between breaths. Pause, briefly holding your breath as you switch fingers at the end of inhalation and pause at the end of exhalation before inhaling again. One way to ensure evenness of breath and breath retention, is to breathe in and out to a count of 4 or 6 and hold between breaths for half the time, say for a count of 2 if inhale and exhale for a count of 4.

NOTE: If you have high blood pressure only retain the breath after exhalation. If you have low blood pressure, only retain the breath after inhalation.

Full Yogic Breath

This technique encourages fuller use of the diaphragm in breathing, providing a massage to the internal organs and improving circulation of blood and lymph.

STARTING POSITION: With hands resting on thighs and breathing through nose:

» Inhale, filling first your abdomen, then expanding your ribcage and chest three-dimensionally, then finally fill your upper chest without raising or straining your shoulders.

» Exhale in a relaxed manner, slightly contracting your abdominal muscles toward the end of exhalation to assist in emptying your lungs of air.

This completes one round of a Full Yogic Breath. Repeat 2–10 rounds.

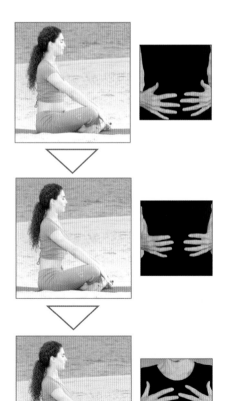

AGNI SARA
Fire Breath

The Fire Breath is a technique that 'fans the fire' of the abdominal area and generates heat and an internal energy source in the core of the body that radiates out to feed the rest of the body. This breathing technique can have a fat-burning effect over time. It also promotes healthy circulation throughout the body and a healthy glow of the skin.

OPTION FOR ARMS WHEN IN A SITTING POSITION: Raise arms to point diagonally upward, palms facing forward, with thumb pointing upwards and rest of fingers curled in to palm.

INSTRUCTION: Use short, relatively fast breaths through your nose, initiated from your abdomen and evenly timed on inhalation and exhalation.

» On inhalation, relax the abdomen allowing it to expand slightly as air is inhaled through the nose.

» On exhalation, sharply pull your navel towards your spine pressing the air out through your nose. Exhalation blows the air out of your nose in a short puff.

» Continue for approximately 20 seconds to a minute or up to 3 minutes when you are an experienced practitioner of this technique.

NOTE: For beginners, if you feel you need a break after a few fire breaths, pause to take one or two deep breaths before continuing. For example, you can split up the breaths to take 8 breaths then one or two deep breaths and repeat in this manner as you build your stamina for this technique.

CAUTION: The fire breath should not leave you feeling hyperventilated when practised correctly. If you do feel yourself getting lightheaded, stop and hang forwards over your legs to take a few breaths to recover. You can also take hold of your feet or place your hands on your head as you hang forward, which can help you regain your feeling of balance more quickly.

BRAHMARI
Bee Breath

The vibration of the hum has a soothing, energising effect on body and mind.

INSTRUCTION: Breathe through your nose, with eyes and mouth closed, humming with each exhalation that is extended as long as you can.

Repeat either A or B, 3–5 times

A With chest tapping: As hum you each exhale, tap all over chest area with both hands (using fists or fingers). Tap front and back of chest, wherever you can reach. This has a lung stimulating effect.

B While lying on back in Savasana.
This technique helps to counteract tension accumulation in the jaw, face and throat.

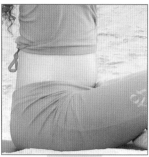

Inhale

Exhale

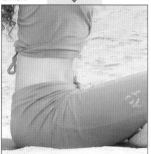

A.

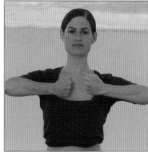

B.

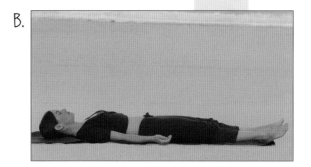

SIMHASANA
The Lion

» Inhale tightening facial muscles, closing eyes tightly and pursing lips.
» Exhale with eyes opened wide and squinting up to look towards the midpoint between your brows. At the same time, open your mouth wide and stick your tongue out while reaching arms and hands downwards over your knees towards the ground with fingers spread. Hold for 2 or 3 breaths.

Inhale

Exhale

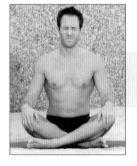 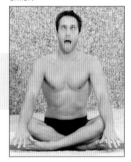

OHM SOUND

This technique has a deeply calming effect on body and mind. Say the word 'ohm' on a long exhalation. Repeat 3 times.

BANDHA
Energy seals, locks or directors

A bandha involves contracting or holding certain body areas. It serves to seal or lock in and redirect subtle energy generated during the practice of Yoga postures and breathing. The effect is to concentrate energy in certain areas of the body, so nourishing the body tissues. Bandha are found to preserve youthfulness and promote vitality.

Bandha can be applied on their own or while holding certain Yoga postures. Instruction is included in chapter 7, for when to apply the locks during the Yoga sessions.

Bandha have been organised into three groups for convenience, guiding you to combine them in practice. They are referred to as lock set #1, 2 and 3.

Lock sets #1 and 2 can be applied on their own or while executing certain Yoga postures. They can also be used with breath retention where specified, at the end of inhalation or exhalation. When retaining breath hold the Bandha for as long as you feel comfortable to hold your breath. Then release your breath and the Bandha together.

A Lock set #1:
Mula Bandha with 'zip lock'.

Mula Bandha involves contracting your perineum, which is the pelvic floor muscles. The effectiveness of this seal is enhanced, and can be easier for beginner practitioners to find, when what is referred to here as the 'zip-lock' seal is also applied. The 'zip-lock' involves contracting your lower abdominal muscles from pubic bone to navel, as if pulling up an internal zip in the core of your body from pubic bone to navel. The effect of this Bandha is to raise energy upwards from the hips to the upper body. It naturally encourages extension of the lower back area supporting spinal elongation from the lower spine in postures. While holding this Bandha in postures, use the Ujjayi breath, breathing mainly into chest area, expanding ribcage three-dimensionally.

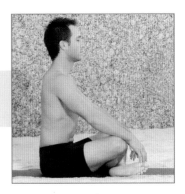

B Lock set #2:
Mula Bandha and Jalandhara Bandha.

This lock set involves application of Lock set #1, with addition of sealing energy in at the level of the neck, directing energy to be concentrated in the torso area. The neck lock involves tucking your chin into your chest, aiming your chin in towards the indent between your collarbones at the top of your chest. This elongates the back of the neck.

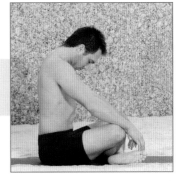

C Lock set #3:
Mula Bandha, Jalandhara Bandha and Uddiyana Bandha.

To be applied while holding breath at the end of exhalation. It involves applying the locks of lock set #2 with addition of pulling your abdomen in towards your spine as if scooping your abdomen up under your ribs to hollow out your abdominal area. This full abdominal contraction is called Uddiyana Bandha. Hold for as long as you are able. Then relax and take a few deep breaths.

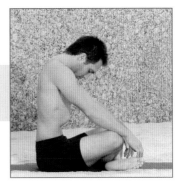

SAVASANA
The Corpse Pose

INSTRUCTION: Lie flat on your back on the ground with legs extended. Legs are a comfortable distance apart and relaxed. Arms rest on the ground at your sides, a comfortable distance from your body, palms up. Check that your body is symmetrical and that the back of your neck is extended along the ground in a comfortable position. Eyes are closed.

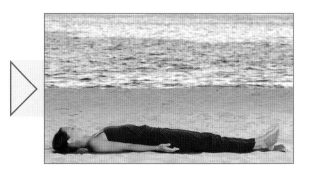

TIMING: Rest in this position for a minimum of 2–5 minutes at the end of a Yoga session or at any time you wish for a replenishing rest.

Allow yourself to surrender your weight into the ground as you relax.

To recover, take a deep breath stretching your arms and legs in opposite directions. Then curl your body to lie on your right side for a breath or few before moving into a sitting position.

Body Stretch with Raised Hips

STARTING POSITION: Start lying on your back with arms extended overhead, resting on the ground alongside your head. Arms and legs are extended in opposite directions. Feet are lightly flexed.

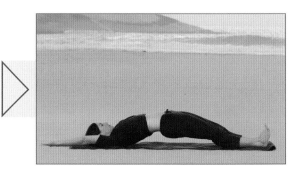

INSTRUCTION: Keeping arms and legs extended raise your hips upwards pressing down through your heels to assist in raising your hips. The weight of your body rests between shoulders and heels with chin naturally in position close to chest.

Sway hips from side to side a few times.

To end, return to lie flat on your back.

APANASANA
Wind-relieving Position

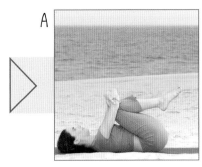

STARTING POSITION: Start lying on your back with legs together and knees bent in over your abdomen. This posture is helpful to digestion.

A Hug your knees in over your abdomen, arms crossed over your knees. Hold for 2–5 breaths or more if desired. Feel breath filling into lower back and hip area with lower back pressed into ground.

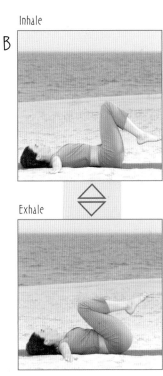

Inhale

B DYNAMIC VERSION: Place arms on the ground reaching out to sides at shoulder height. Knees are held in over your abdomen and bent with heels towards hips. Flex or point your feet and maintain this throughout. Apply lock set #1 (p. 53) and hold throughout. On exhalation contract your lower abdomen, drawing your knees in towards your chest, raising your hips off the ground slightly. On inhalation release abdominal contraction, so returning to starting position. Repeat 8 times.

Exhale

C DYNAMIC VERSION WITH KNEE/LEG CIRCLING: With arms and legs in starting position as for dynamic version B, draw circles in the air with your knees so that your lower back area receives a massage. Move knees together over to the right, to feel pressure under right side of back, and continue to draw knees in over abdomen toward chest. Then, continue to circle the knees over to the left so pressure is felt under the left side of the back, then return to the starting position with the lower spine in contact with the ground. Apply lock set #1 (p. 53) and hold throughout. Repeat in the same direction 2–4 times, inhaling as knees are pulled in to chest, exhaling as knees move away. Then repeat circles in opposite direction.

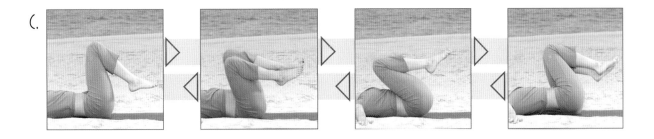

Rolling Ball

The rolling ball can help break down excess fat accumulation in the torso area, particularly on the back, which receives a massage. It also gives a squeeze to the internal organs in the contracted position, promoting health and a healthy spinal column.

STARTING POSITION: Lie on your back with knees bent and held in over your abdomen, hands holding behind your knees.

INSTRUCTION: Round your spine, tucking chin in towards chest. Initiate a backwards and forwards rocking motion, inhaling to rock backwards, exhaling to rock forwards. Your legs can assist you to gain momentum by kicking slightly overhead each time you inhale to rock backwards. Rock more or less 8 times.

Options A or B allow you to adjust the rolling ball action relative to your spinal flexibility:

A Use small rocking motion with hips and upper back rising alternately, keeping spine round with chin tucked in to chest.

B For a flexible spine, inhale to rock backwards so that knees are brought overhead and weight of body rests on shoulders. Exhale to rock forwards all the way up to a sitting position. Spine remains rounded with chin tucked into chest throughout.

A.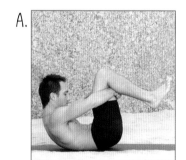

B.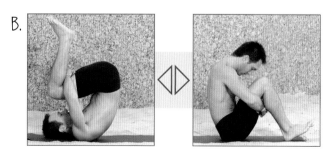

JATHARA PARIVARTANASANA
Spinal Twists

STARTING POSITION: Lie on your back with knees hugged in over your abdomen as for Apanasana position A.

INSTRUCTION: Then, keeping legs in position, extend arms out to sides on the ground with palms down.

Particularly breathe into the chest area, expanding this area on inhalation while holding spinal twists. For both A and B, hold for 3 to 8 breaths in twist each side.

A Exhaling, lower legs to the right, keeping legs together. Aim to keep both shoulders and upper chest in contact with the ground as much as possible. Place right hand over left knee to support and stabilise the position. Hold in this position. To recover: Inhale as return to centred starting position. Repeat to other side.

B Extend legs along the ground ahead of you, keeping legs together. Feet are pointed or semi pointed, with balls of feet reaching forward and toes flexed. On an exhalation, keeping both legs extended, initiate a twist to the right from your hips, sliding your left leg over to the right side to rest on the ground pointing to the right, raising the left leg only as high as you can. Maintain contact of both shoulders with the ground. Hold in this twisting stretch.

TO RECOVER: Inhale as return to centred starting position. Repeat to the other side.

A.

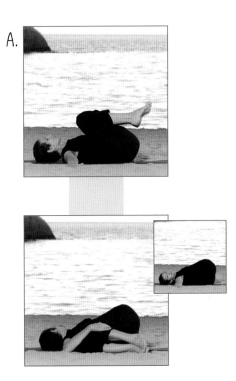

B.

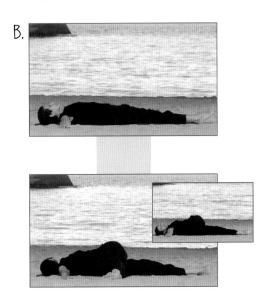

Dynamic Leg Raises

STARTING POSITION: Lying on back with knees hugged in over abdomen, legs together. Coordinate arm and leg movements in moving between A and B, as well as coordinating breath with smooth movement.

A Inhaling, raise arms, placing them on the ground above your head, with arms extended and parallel. Legs bend in over abdomen, with feet flexed.

B Exhaling, with lower back pressed into ground, extend legs upwards to vertical position, until stretched as far as you can, with feet flexed, soles of feet facing upwards. At the same time, arms follow a semicircular pathway, raising them up in front of you and lowering them down to your sides.

Move between A and B 4–8 times.

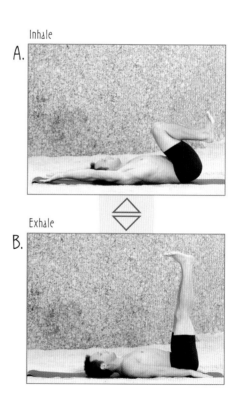

Inhale

A.

Exhale

B.

Leg Walking

STARTING POSITION FOR A AND B: Lie on your back, with legs together, extended vertically upwards (or slightly bent if need be) and parallel, with feet flexed.

A Extend arms along ground reaching out to sides in line with shoulders, palms down. Open and close legs 4–8 times.

B Raise arms to point upward parallel to raised legs. Walk legs and arms forwards and backwards in a scissor-like motion, with arms walking in opposition to legs. Press lower and middle of spine into ground throughout. Repeat scissor motion 8–16 times, where each time you move, you use short, sharp exhalations, pressing navel towards the ground to force air out nose with each exhalation, like the fire breath with short inhalations and exhalations of equal length. To end, hug knees in over abdomen and hold for a few breaths.

A.

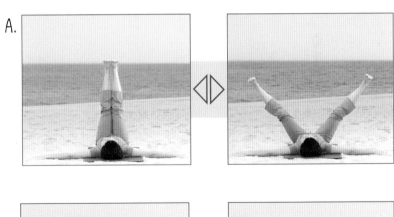

B.

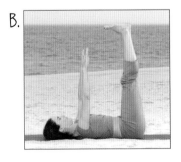
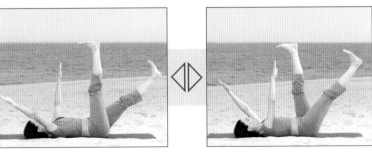

SETU BANDHA SARVANGASANA
The Little Bridge

STARTING POSITION: Lie on your back with legs bent, parallel and hip distance apart, with knees pointing upward, and soles of feet on the ground. Arms are on the ground at your sides, palms down. Press your lower back into the ground on an exhalation to initiate moving into the position.

INSTRUCTION: Then, as you inhale, stand into your feet to assist you in raising your hips upwards gradually, peeling your spine off the ground vertebra for vertebra until the weight of your body rests between your shoulders and your feet with hips raised as high as you can. Feel your skin stretching between your knees and shoulders with chest raised up towards chin. Hold for 5–8 breaths.

TO RECOVER: On exhalation reverse the spine-peeling action, smoothly rolling down, vertebra for vertebra until your hips reach the ground. Feel the massage to your spinal column as you roll up and down your spine.

URDHVA DHANURASANA
The Full Bridge

In some schools the full bridge is referred to as Chakrasana. It is an advanced posture not to be attempted by beginners until well experienced in other back bending postures.

INSTRUCTION: Start from the Little Bridge position with hips raised. Bring your hands alongside your head with elbows raised and palms flat on the ground with fingers pointing towards your shoulders. Move into the full bridge in stages.

First inhale to raise chest upwards, supported by hands and feet on the ground, to position with crown of head placed on the ground. On next inhale press up into the full bridge, raising hips upwards as you inflate your chest and stand securely into both feet. Arms extend and legs remain slightly bent. Weight is shared evenly between hands and feet. Look out or down to the ground between your hands. Hold for 5–8 breaths.

TO RECOVER: Reverse the path you took moving in to the position. Then use counterposture such as Apanasana (p. 55) and Pascimottanasana (p. 71), as specified.

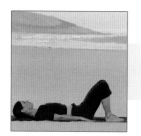
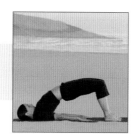

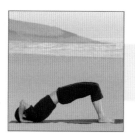
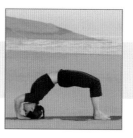
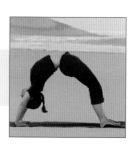

SARVANGASANA
The Shoulder Stand

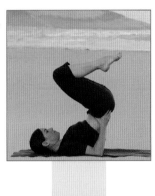

STARTING POSITION: Start lying on your back with knees hugged in over abdomen. Check that your spine and neck are centred as you lie on the ground. For holding, use position A or C for 5–8 breaths.

A **VIPARITA KARANI:** Place hands under hips and round your spine, swinging your legs overhead. Rest your hips into your hands, supported by your elbows on the ground. Legs extend diagonally upward, as close to vertical as comfortably possible. Feet are pointed or half pointed with balls of feet reaching upward, toes flexed.

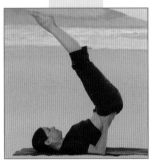

B **VERSION WITH LEG KICKING:** In position A, flex feet and alternate legs in a relatively fast kicking motion with heels aiming to kick your buttocks each time. Continue approximately 16 to 20 times or more.

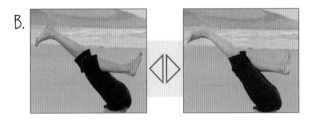

C **SARVANGASANA—THE SHOULDER STAND:** From position A, bring your hips forward as you raise your legs and feet vertically upward so that shoulders, hips and feet are in one line. Feet are extended upward with toes flexed so that the balls of your feet are the highest point reaching upward. If you can, adjust the position of your elbows on the ground to bring elbows closer together towards parallel position for better support. Also position your hands as high on your upper back (as close to your shoulders) as you can. Hold in this position.

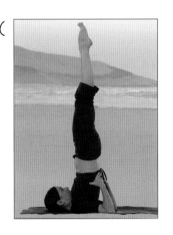

TO RECOVER: Slowly roll down your spine vertebra for vertebra until you are lying back down on the ground. Your hands support this descent. In the sessions there is the option to move directly into Halasana—The Plough from the shoulder stand position.

HALASANA
The Plough

INSTRUCTION: From supported shoulder stand position or from position lying on your back with knees bent, reach legs and feet overhead then down towards the ground, keeping legs extended. Flex feet and if your feet touch the ground, place toes curled under on ground.

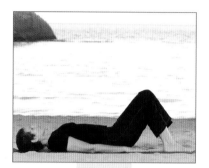

ARM POSITION: Place arms on the ground at your sides, palms down or with fingers interlocked, hands palm to palm, arms extended along the ground pointing away from you. Feel two-way stretch between heels of extended legs reaching in one direction and arms reaching in the opposite direction. If your feet do not touch the ground, remain in position with hands supporting hips.
  Hold for 5 breaths.

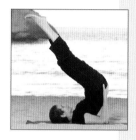
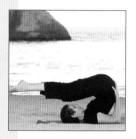

TO RECOVER: Place your hands on your hips or lower back for support as you slowly roll down your spine vertebra for vertebra until you are lying back down on the ground. Legs remain extended until spine rests on the ground, then bend your knees to slide feet out along ground to extended position. Alternatively you can move in to the Rolling Ball (p. 56) rocking a few times to recover to a sitting position.

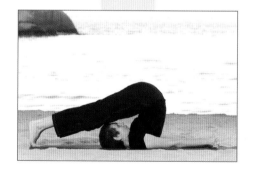

MATSYANA
The Fish

STARTING POSITION: Lie on your back with legs extended, held together and parallel. Feet are pointed, with toes flexed so balls of feet reach forward. Place hands palms down under your upper legs or buttocks, wherever they reach with arms extended, so you are lying on your hands.

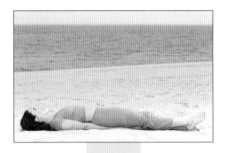

A SIMPLE VERSION: On inhalation, arch your spine, inflating and raising your chest upwards so your upper back arches and chest lifts up towards your chin. Elbows press down into the ground as your arms bend to support the position.

A.

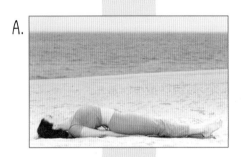

B From position A, on inhalation, raise your chest higher, shifting the position of your head to place the crown of your head on the ground so that your spine is in a full arch from tailbone to top of neck and you are looking out behind you. Adjust the position of your elbows to be closer together if possible, to assist in further opening shoulders and chest.
  Hold position A or B for 3–5 breaths.

B.

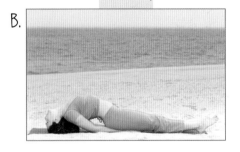

TO RECOVER: Slowly return to starting position lying back on ground.

Dynamic Sit-up Versions

STARTING POSITION: Lie on your back with legs together and extended with feet flexed.

  For all options, repeat 4–8 times, dynamically alternating exhale as you sit up and inhale as you lie back down.

A Bend arms to place hands under upper neck where neck meets skull, with elbows resting on the ground pointing out to sides. Inhale extending your spine. Exhale as you raise your shoulders, upper torso and head off the ground as high as you can without straining, looking toward your toes. Press your navel down toward the ground as you sit up, keeping lower back pressed into the ground. Elbows remain open to the sides. Avoid straining your neck; only sit up as far as the strength of your abdominal muscles allow. Inhale as you lower your spine back down to the ground.

B Sit-ups into forward bend with legs apart: Extend arms overhead to rest on ground alongside head, with legs apart in a straddle position, feet flexed. Inhale reaching legs and arms in opposite directions. Exhaling sit up to reach your hands towards your heels, on the inner sides of your flexed feet. Inhale to lie back down to starting position with legs open.

C Sit-ups into forward bend with legs together: As for version B, with legs together. Inhale as stretch arms and legs in opposite directions. Exhale sitting all the way up to forward bend over extended legs with hands reaching to feet. Then inhale reversing motion to lie back down again with arms stretched upwards alongside head.

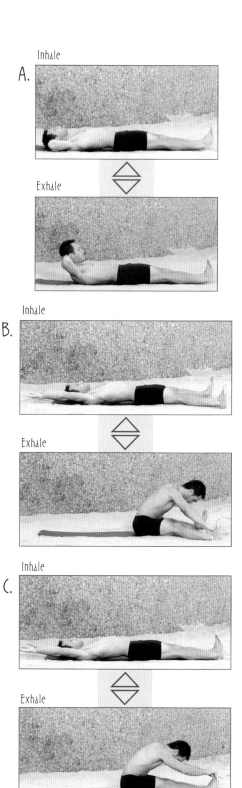

Dynamic Body Curls

STARTING POSITION: Lie on your back, with legs and arms extended in opposite directions.

» Inhale stretching arms and legs in opposite directions.

» Exhaling, curl your body sideways to the left, sliding along the ground to bring left elbow towards left knee, to curl body into foetal position lying on your left side.

» Inhaling, uncurl your body, returning to starting position lying on your back with arms and legs extending in opposite directions.

» Exhaling, curl to right side.

» Repeat 2 or 3 times to each side alternately.

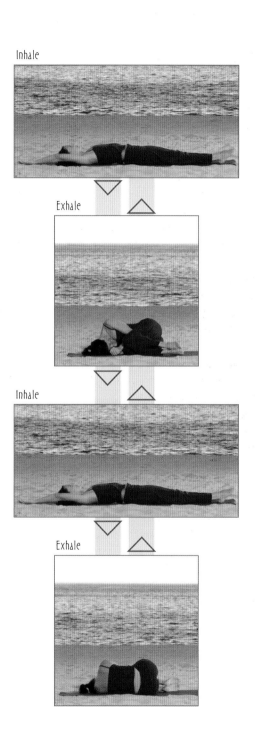

Inhale

Exhale

Inhale

Exhale

Preparatory series for DHANURASANA (The Bow), including BHUJANGASANA (The Cobra) and SALABHASANA (The Locust)

STARTING POSITION: Lie on your front with arms at your sides. Legs are together, parallel and squeezed together, with feet extended. Tighten your buttock (gluteal) muscles to assist in reaching your legs away from you. Maintain this energetic leg extension with legs together for all the following exercises unless otherwise specified.

A BHUJANGASANA—THE COBRA, SUPPORTED VERSION: Inhale to raise upper body off the ground using the strength of your back muscles. Place your elbows on the ground, with arms parallel to each other, directly under shoulders. Head and eyes look down to the ground between your hands or, if your spine is flexible, look out in front of you. Feel spine long in this position with head reaching forward and up, and shoulders pressed down so body weight is 'lifted out' of shoulders. Hold in this position for 3–8 breaths, inflating your chest on inhalation and feeling how the position naturally stretches the skin across your abdomen.

B WITH HANDS UNDER FOREHEAD: Place backs of hands under forehead with elbows bent and pointing out to sides. Raise upper body and head, with hands remaining against forehead, elbows pointing out to sides. Shoulders press down into your back so that your neck is long. Hold for 3–8 breaths, inflating your chest on inhalation.

C SALABHASANA—THE LOCUST: Place hands in fists under your legs in your groin area. In this position, place forehead on the ground or turn head to side with cheek resting on ground. On inhalation, raise both legs to reach back and up with legs extended and pointed. Legs remain squeezed together. Hands help to prop your legs up in the position, also helping you raise your legs up higher. Hold for 3–8 breaths.

D WITH HANDS CLASPED BEHIND BACK: Clasp hands behind back with fingers interlocked, palms together, rolling shoulders open to expand your chest. Inhale raising upper body with head looking down or out in front of you, and legs as for the locust, keeping legs squeezed together and feet pointed. Arms raise to reach back towards feet. Hold for 3–8 breaths inflating your chest on inhalation to allow you to raise your upper body further into the back-bending position.

E DHANURASANA—THE BOW: With arms at sides, bend both legs, bringing feet in towards hips with legs parallel and hip distance apart. Reach your arms back to take hold of your ankles. Inhaling, raise upper body, arms and legs into Bow position with your weight balancing on your hips and lower abdomen. Hold for 5–8 breaths. If you feel comfortable to do so, you can use a gentle rock backwards and forwards in the position a few times before holding. This gives a massage to the abdominal area.

F 'SWIMMING' VERSIONS: Start lying on front, with arms extended out in front of you alongside head, reaching forward while resting on the ground. Legs are extended and squeezed together with arms and legs reaching in opposite directions. Inhaling, tighten into your buttock muscles to support raising upper body and legs so weight rests on your abdomen and hips. Arms extend forward parallel to ground with arms and legs reaching in opposite directions. (i) Open and close legs 4–8 times while remaining in position with body raised. Head looks forward or down towards the ground. (ii) Reaching arms forward raised in position parallel to ground, with legs extended. Arms remain still in this position. Head looks forward or down towards the ground. Kick legs up and down behind you as if swimming, keeping legs and feet extended. Repeat 8–16 times. Then repeat (i) and (ii) again.

A.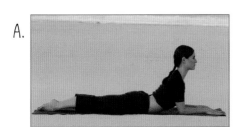

B.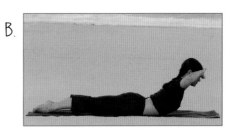

C.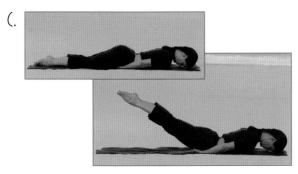
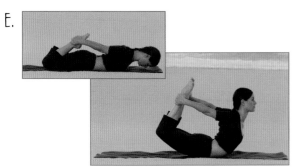

D.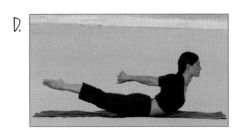

E.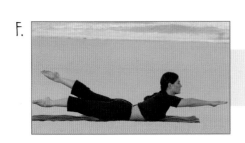

F.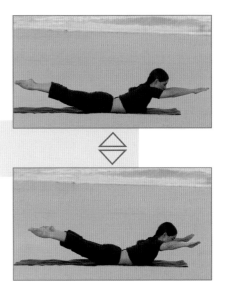

Lower Back Mobilising Exercises

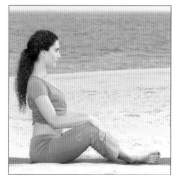

Inhale

STARTING POSITION: Sit with soles of feet together, legs forming a wide diamond shape with heels a comfortable distance away from hips. Breathe through nose throughout.

INSTRUCTION: Inhaling, tilt pelvis forward so that the lower back arches.

Exhaling, tilt pelvis backward, so that lower back rounds.

Inhalation and exhalation are equal in length. Move between inhalation and exhalation at a comfortable pace. Aim toward fairly swift, short, even breaths, as for the Fire Breath (p. 50) with a loose, shaking-out quality to the movement.

Carry out 8–20 or more times at a speed comfortable to you, not too fast, not too slow.

OPTIONAL: Follow above exercise with shaking hips from side to side on the ground while in sitting position, as if shaking up the contents of your pelvic bowl. Repeat a few times, feeling a loosening into the hip and lower back area.

Exhale

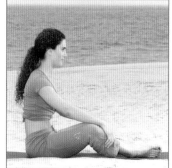

Upper Body Swing

STARTING POSITION: Sit with legs crossed. Sit evenly on both hips with spine extended as central axis.

A Place hands on your shoulders, raising elbows to shoulder height, pointing out to sides. Breathe through your nose. Eyes are closed. Inhaling swing shoulders and upper body to twist to the left, with neck and head naturally following your upper body twist to the left. Exhaling, swing to the right. Swing 8 or more times to each side, coordinating breath with movement. Breathing is at the pace of a comfortable swinging motion.

B Continue to swing as for A with hands clasped behind neck, elbows open and pointing out to sides. Swing 8–16 or more times to each side.

C Arm stretch-up with locks as counter-posture after A and B: Interlock fingers above head, palms facing up. Stretch arms upwards, pushing up with hands as you take a deep inhale and hold breath while applying lock set #2 (p. 53). Then exhale and hold breath at end of exhale while applying lock set #3 (p. 53). Then take a deep breath, relaxing arms.

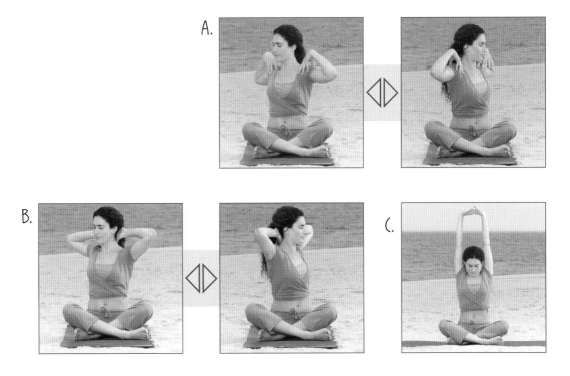

JANU SIRSASANA
Head to Knee Pose

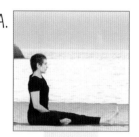

A **STARTING POSITION:** Sit with spine upright, legs extended, together and parallel with knees pulled up into thighs, and feet flexed. Bend left leg, so knee points out to side, placing sole of foot up against right inner thigh. Place left hand on left ankle to help bring this foot as close in to groin as possible. Right arm rests on ground at your side. Check that you are sitting evenly on both hips, with hips and shoulders facing squarely to the front.

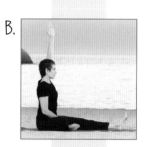

OPTIONAL FOOT WARM-UP: Circle the ankle and foot of extended leg 3 times in each direction.

B On inhalation, raise right arm sideways and up, to reach vertically upward, alongside your head, palm facing to the left.

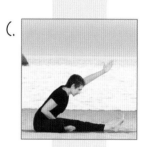

C Bend forward from hips as far as you can keeping spine and leg extended and foot flexed, with arm reaching diagonally upward. Then lower your right hand to take hold of your right ankle or foot wherever you can reach.

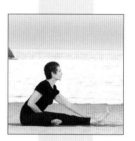

D Inhale deeply then exhale into full forward bend, bringing head towards knee or foot with spine extending forwards. Both arms now hold foot or leg, wherever you can reach with elbows lowered down to the ground to help you deepen your forward bend and relax your shoulders in the position. Shoulders are symmetrical and pressed down so neck and spine are long. Hold for 5 breaths.

TO RECOVER: Reverse path taken into posture, returning to starting position. Repeat with left leg extended.

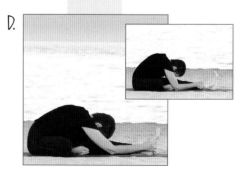

PASCIMOTTANASANA
Sitting Forward Bend

A STARTING POSITION: Sit with spine upright, legs extended, together and parallel with knees pulled up into thighs, and feet flexed. Place fingertips on the ground alongside and slightly behind your hips, with elbows bent and pulled backward to open shoulders and chest. This position encourages sitting position with chest open and spine long.

B On inhalation, raise both arms sideways and up to parallel position reaching up alongside head, palms facing each other, head looks forward.

NOTE: Keep shoulders held down so there is distance between shoulders and ears. Feel two-way stretch between hips and upper body, as arms and upper body reach upwards and hips reach downwards into the ground creating space in your waist. Allow chest to raise or inflate slightly to free arms to reach upwards more easily.

C On exhalation, bend forward from your hips as far as you can, keeping spine, arms and legs extended, with spine and arms reaching diagonally upward. Head remains in line with spine, eyes looking down in front of you.

D Then lower hands to legs to take hold of calves or ankles or feet, depending on how far you can reach.

E Move into the full forward bend, with spine extended as much as possible, reaching head forward then down towards legs as you move into the position. Ease elbows down toward the ground. Hold for 5–8 breaths.

TO RECOVER: Reverse path taken into posture, returning to starting position.

A.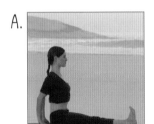

B.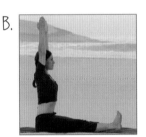

C.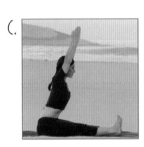

D.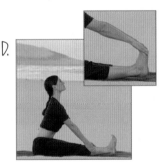

E.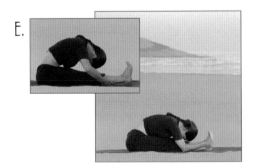

Half Bridge

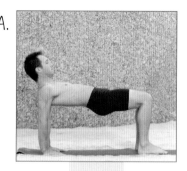

A.

STARTING POSITION: sitting with legs extended out in front of you. Part legs to hip distance apart. Spine is upright. Hands rest on the ground at your sides, with arms parallel, hands flat on the ground and fingers pointing forwards.

A HALF BRIDGE STATIC VERSION (REFER TO PICTURES FOR B THEN A): On exhalation, bending your knees to stand into your feet and bending your elbows, move hips towards heels, shifting weight to rest between hands and feet with hips suspended off the ground. Legs and feet are parallel. Eyes look out in front of you with chin tucked in toward chest. On inhalation, continue to raise hips and chest upwards, standing into your feet and extending your arms, aiming for a table-top position, with weight shared between hands and feet. Either keep your head with chin tucked into chest, or if you feel comfortable to do so, hang your head back, stretching out your throat area, with eyes looking out behind you. Pointers: Keep shoulders pressed down and open, with arms lengthened, so that neck and upper back are relatively free. Also check that legs and feet remain parallel. Hold for 5 breaths.

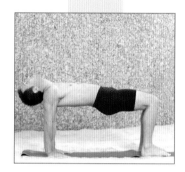

B DYNAMIC VERSION: From starting position, sitting upright with legs extended, inhale moving into position A, with head to navel or looking out behind you. Then exhale returning to starting position. Repeat 8 times or more.

C WITH PULSING AND LEG RAISING: Start in position A with hips raised, eyes looking to navel. (i) Place left ankle over right knee with left knee opened out to side. Pulse your hips up and down with a small motion so you mainly feel the work in your buttock muscles. Repeat 8 times. Switch legs to repeat. (ii) Extend right leg with foot pointing forward and resting on the ground, keeping hips as raised as possible. Raise and lower your right leg 4–8 times. Repeat with left leg.

D Half bridge as inclined plank with legs extended: Start in position A and extend both legs so feet rest on ground, legs parallel and held together, feet pointing forward and as close to flat on the ground as your feet will allow. Keep hips raised as high as you can. Head is eased backward so looking out behind you, or if uncomfortable for your neck, remain with chin to chest, looking towards navel. Hold for 3–8 breaths.

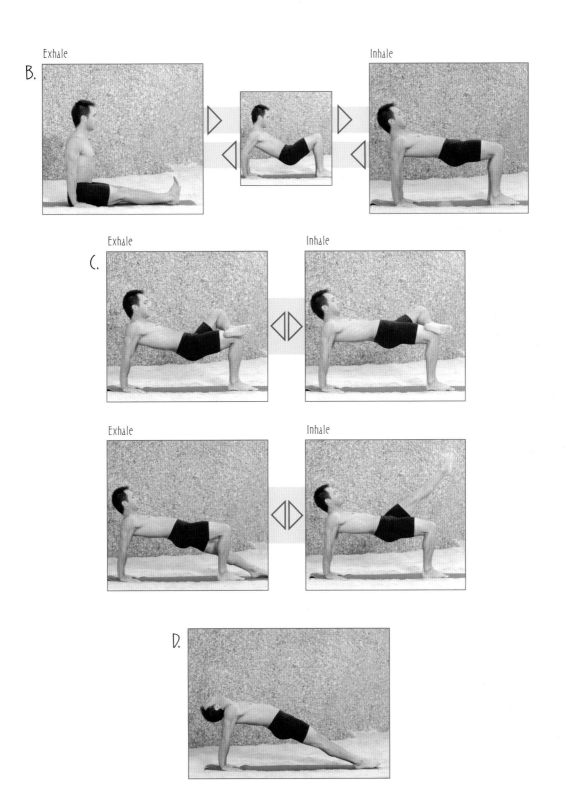

B.

Exhale

Inhale

C.

Exhale

Inhale

Exhale

Inhale

D.

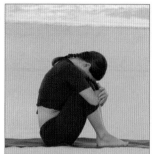

A.

PARIPURNA NAVASANA
The Boat

A Sit with spine upright, legs bent, hugging knees into chest with feet flat or up on balls of feet.

B Take hold of outer side of both ankles with same-side hands. Lean back slightly as you raise your legs diagonally upward, extending your legs as much as you can with hands supporting legs. Weight balances on hips. Keep spine extended as you find your balance. Balance for 3–8 breaths.

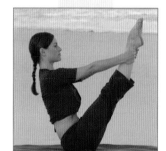

B.

C From position A or B, reach arms forward to position parallel to the ground, palms facing in towards each other. Keep spine well extended and neck long, with chin slightly lowered in towards chest. Eyes look forward. Legs can be slightly bent if need be. Balance for 3–8 breaths. Then return to starting position hugging knees into chest.

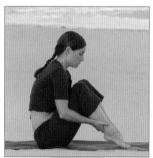

D Start sitting with knees hugged into chest. Open knees as take hold of inside of soles of feet. Extend and raise your legs, opening legs out to the sides. Find your balance on your hips with spine and legs extending.

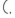
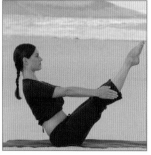

C.

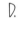
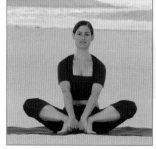

D.

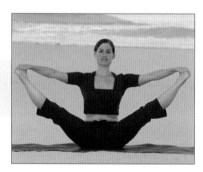

BADDHA KONASANA
The Butterfly

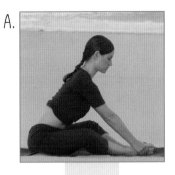

A **SIMPLE BUTTERFLY VERSION:** Sit with soles of feet together, heels a comfortable distance away from your hips, forming a diamond shape, knees as close to the ground as possible. Hold feet as you relax torso and head in to forward bend over legs. Elbows open out to knees. Hold for 3–8 breaths or more.

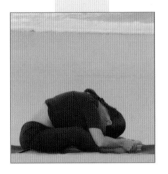

B Another option for arms: Place palms together, then interlock thumbs in the palms of your hands so fingertips remain touching. Reach arms forward along the ground. Head hangs forward between arms.
To recover, uncurl spine to upright, bringing head up last.

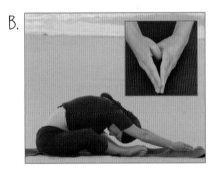

(BADDHA KONASANA—THE BUTTERFLY: Start sitting in simple Butterfly position with soles of feet together and spine extended upright. Draw heels as close in to your hips as possible. Knees press down towards the ground. Take hold of your feet with your hands and bend forward over your legs, bringing your head towards your feet and opening your elbows out to the sides. Hold for 3–5 breaths or more.

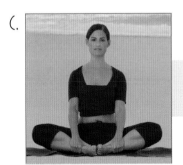

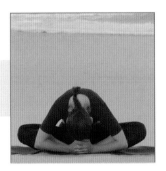

UPAVISTA KONASANA
The Straddle

 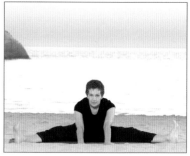

STARTING POSITION: sitting evenly on both hips, with legs extended out to sides as far as you can, knees pulled up into thighs and feet flexed so legs are well extended. Maintain this leg position throughout. Hands rest on the ground in front of you as you sit with spine upright.

A Move into forward bend with hands supporting position on ground. Keep spine as extended as you can. If you can, move further into forward bend, either placing hands or elbows on the ground, or holding your feet.

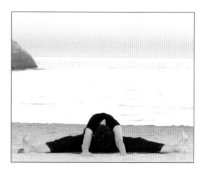

Hold for 5 breaths. Then return to upright position.

B With side bend: Start sitting upright. Bend sideways to the right with left arm reaching overhead to the right. Right arm is either in front of you on the ground, or you can rest right hand on right leg, or place right hand on the ground behind your right leg—whichever is more comfortable. Head and eyes face forward. Hold for 2 or 3 breaths.

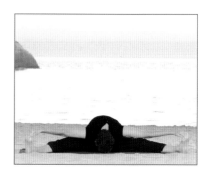

   Then inhale to recover to upright starting position. Repeat to other side.

POINTERS: In side bend sit evenly on both hips, with hips and shoulders facing squarely to the front. Keep legs stretched with feet flexed so you feel a two-way stretch between heel and opposite arm extended overhead.

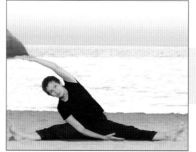 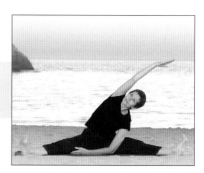

Version of
EKA PADA RAJAKAPOTASANA
The Pigeon

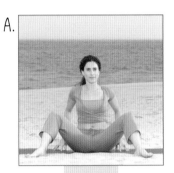

A STARTING POSITION: Sit with spine upright, legs bent and opened out to sides with soles of feet on the ground. Knees point upwards. Hands are placed on the ground behind your hips.

B Twist your hips to the left, lowering your knees toward the ground to point to the left so your body faces the left side.

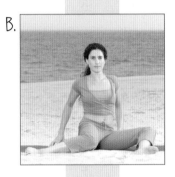

C Bend right leg with foot pointing upwards, and take hold of right ankle in right hand. Left hand remains on the ground at your left side for support. On inhalation, twist your torso and head to look over your left shoulder. Feel stretch across your right thigh and hip. You may need to adjust the position, shifting your right leg further out behind you to find the stretch. Hold for 3–5 breaths each side.

TO RECOVER: Return to centred starting position. Repeat to other side.

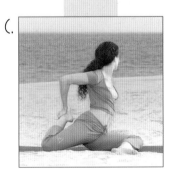

Crossed Leg Forward Stretch

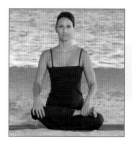
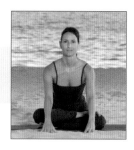

This position gives a stretch to the outer sides of the hip and contributes to lower back comfort and health.

INSTRUCTION: Cross right leg over left, with right ankle over left knee or thigh and right knee opened out to side. Bend forward over legs, feeling stretch to outer side of right hip. Arms rest on your legs or extend forwards with hands resting on the ground for support. Head faces forward or relax into forward bend. Hold for 3–5 breaths. Repeat to other side.

Version of SUPTA VIRASANA

A Start in Vajrasana position sitting on heels with legs together and folded underneath you. Open your feet out to the sides of your hips, shifting your calf muscles out of the way so you can sit between your heels. If you feel strain in your knees, you can either sit on a cushion, or support you weight with your hands for a few breaths to help your body become used to the position over time.

B From position A, if you can, lean back on your elbows behind you.

C If you are able to, lie back bringing your shoulders to the ground, reaching your arms overhead to rest on the ground alongside your head with fingers interlocked, palms facing your head. Keep knees close together and pressing down towards the ground. This position promotes healthy digestion.

Avoid this posture (A, B and C) if you have varicose veins or if you feel strain in your knees.

A.
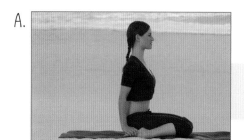

B.
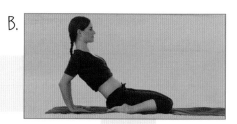

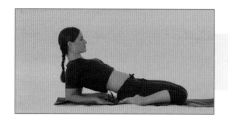

C.
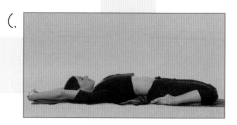

Neck Stretches

STARTING POSITION: Sit in comfortable cross-legged position, with spine upright.

A Hang head forwards, chin to chest with shoulders relaxed. Feel stretch to back of neck. Hold for 2–5 breaths. For added support, you can place your fingers at the back of your neck, wherever it feels best.

B Extend your right arm diagonally down to the ground at your side with hand flexed. Lower your head to the left side, bringing left ear toward left shoulder so feel stretch to the right side of your neck. Hold for 2 breaths. Repeat to other side.

C Neck rolls: Inhale lowering head toward left shoulder, keeping shoulders relaxed as feel stretch to right side of neck. Head faces forward. Then exhale lowering head forward, chin to chest. Then inhale bending neck to right, right ear toward right shoulder so feel stretch to left side of neck. Then exhale lowering head, chin to chest, and inhale returning head to side stretch to the left. Repeat 2–4 times, moving slowly and steadily, coordinating breath and movement.

Eye Exercises

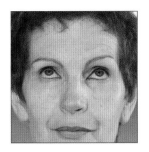

INSTRUCTION: Sit in a comfortable upright position. Circle eyes 3 times in each direction, not too fast, not too slow. Keep eyes in focus throughout. For additional eye exercise, look up and down and side to side a few times, followed by looking up and down to diagonally opposite corners a few times.

To end, hold a steady focus on a point in front of you on the ground for a few breaths.

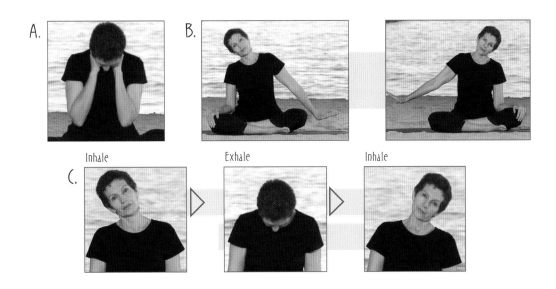

A. B.

Inhale   Exhale   Inhale

C.

ARM STRETCHES

Arm Stretch Series

Sit in a comfortable cross-legged position, or can be done standing. Move through A–E with right arm. Thereafter repeat all with left arm. Then move on to F–I where both arms work together and symmetrically.

A Raise right arm, reaching vertically upwards, fingers pointing upwards, palm facing front. Keep right shoulder held down so there is space between shoulder and ear. Reach over or behind your head with left hand, to take hold of right elbow, supporting right arm. Sway shoulders and chest from side to side a few times.

B From position A, bend right arm at elbow, so palm of right hand rests along spine with fingers pointing downward. Use left hand to ease right elbow behind your head. Take a breath or 2 as you bend upper body over to left side to stretch out under right armpit, then return to centred upright position.

C Bring right arm forward, to extend in front of you, palm up. Bend your hand backwards, palm facing away from you with arm extended, left hand gently pulling back on right fingers to assist the stretch. Hold for a breath. Then bend right wrist and hand up so fingers point upwards, palm facing in toward you and use your left hand to assist giving a stretch to the back side of your wrist, gently easing your palm towards your lower forearm. Hold for a breath.

D Take hold of the outside of your right wrist with left hand and bring right arm across chest to point to left side, approximately at shoulder height, with palm facing back. Bend left arm over right elbow to secure a stretch into your upper right arm and shoulder. Turn head to look over right shoulder, keeping right shoulder pressed down so space between chin and shoulder. Check shoulders are symmetrical. Hold for 2–3 breaths.

E Twist from your waist, around to the left, placing right hand on outside of left thigh with left hand resting on ground behind your spine. Spine is extended and shoulders are symmetrical and pressed down. Look over your left shoulder. Hold for 1–2 deep breaths. To recover, move into a twisting swing from side to side 3 or 4 times, breathing in and out alternately to each side. Arms swing along, slightly bent at the elbows and raised to a comfortable height for ease of swing. Head follows along naturally to look from side to side.

Repeat all to other side. Then move on to F–I.

F Shoulder stretch, hooking fingers behind head, elbows opened out to sides. Hold for 2 breaths inflating chest on inhalation

G Push hands out to sides at shoulder height, hands flexed, palms facing outward. First do two wrist circles in each direction with both hands simultaneously. Then hold position with hands flexed so feel 'nervy' stretch along arm while extending arms out to sides at shoulder height. Hold for 2 breaths.

H Clasp hands behind lower back and extend arms, raising them upwards. Hold for 2 or 3 breaths inflating chest on inhalation

I PRAYER POSE BEHIND BACK: Meet fingertips or palms of hands behind your back in a prayer pose. Hold for 3 breaths.

A.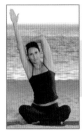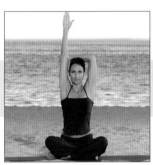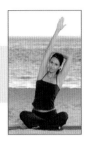

B.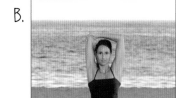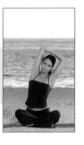

C.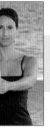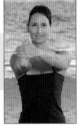

D.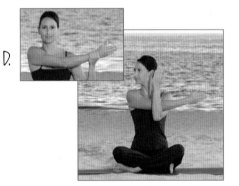

E.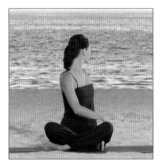

F.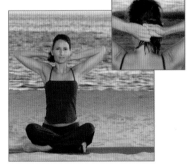

G.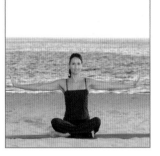

H.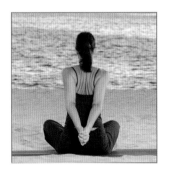

I.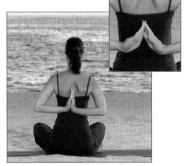

GOMUKHASANA
Cow–Face Posture Arm Position

A Start from position B of the arm stretch series (p. 80–81), with left hand holding right elbow.

B Extend left arm out to left side and bend at elbow to place back of left hand on your back, palm facing out, and reaching up towards left hand. Both hands are placed along spine. Head looks forward with spine and neck upright. Hold in this position or, if you can, hook fingers of left and right hands. Hold for 5 breaths.

Repeat to other side.

C As counterposture, hook fingers behind neck with elbows out to sides, so feel stretch across shoulders and chest. Hold for 2 or 3 breaths, breathing into chest.

KNEELING POSTURES

SUPTA VAJRASANA
The Child's Pose

STARTING POSITION: Sit back on your heels, with legs bent underneath you, rest forward with forehead on the ground. If forehead doesn't reach ground, hang head forward, perhaps placing top of head on ground.

A Arms at sides, with shoulders relaxed over knees.

or

B Extend arms to reach out in front of you, elbows and hands rest on the ground.

Rest for 5 breaths or more.

A.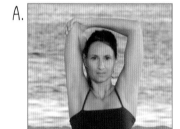

B.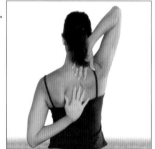

C.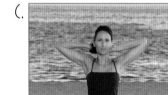

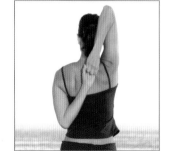

A.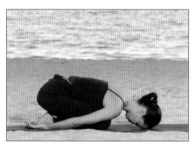

B.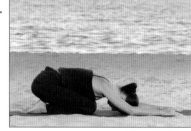

BIDALASANA
Cat Stretch

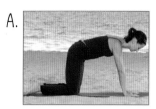
A.

A Start on all fours, with knees under hips and hands under shoulders.

B DYNAMIC CAT STRETCH: Inhale hollowing spine, lowering navel towards the ground, raising hips, chest and head upward. Then exhale, rounding your spine, initiating from navel area, tucking hips and head under so eyes look towards hips. Repeat 4–6 times, coordinating breath with smooth movement.

Inhale   Exhale

B.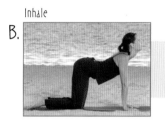

C DYNAMIC VERSION BETWEEN CHILD'S POSE AND COBRA: Start on all fours with wide base (hands on ground ahead of shoulders) and feet with toes curled under. Inhale bringing hips forwards, upper body moving forward between arms as bring hips to the ground and raise chest and head upward. Exhaling, raise your hips to sit back on your heels, moving in to the Child's Pose with arms extended, hands and forehead on the ground. Move between the Cobra and Child's Pose position 3–5 times, coordinating breath with movement.

Inhale   Exhale

C.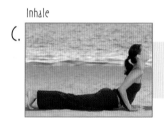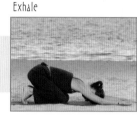

D CAT STRETCH WITH LEG EXTENSIONS: Co-ordinate leg motion with Dynamic Cat Stretch A. Inhaling, hollow spine as extend right leg behind you with leg and foot stretched, feeling two-way stretch between head and foot. Exhaling, rounding spine, drawing right knee in towards forehead. Repeat 3–5 times, moving smoothly between inhaling to extend leg, exhaling to fold leg in to forehead. Then repeat to other side.

Inhale

D.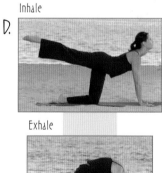

Exhale

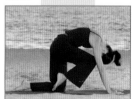

ADHO MUKHA SVANASANA
Dog Stretch

A Start on all fours with wide base (hands on ground ahead of shoulders).

B Curl toes under then raise hips upwards to form an inverted V shape with arms extended, hands flat on the ground and legs extending as much as you can, with heels pressing down towards the ground. Weight is evenly distributed between hands and feet. Head is between arms with spine long, chest aiming towards the ground, ears next to upper arms. Hold for 5 breaths.

C WITH LEG EXTENSION: Starting in the Dog Stretch position B, raise right leg to reach up behind you as high as you can with foot pointed. Keep your head between your arms as for position B or look toward your hands in the position. Hold for 3–5 breaths. Then repeat with left leg raised.

A.

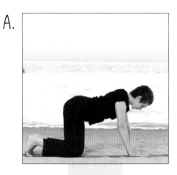

B.

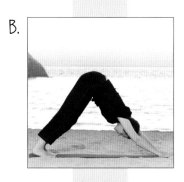

C.

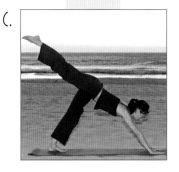

PLANK POSE Versions

A CHATURANGASANA—THE PLANK: Start on all fours. Step your legs out behind you, toes curled under, with legs together, forming a straight line from heels to head. Hands are positioned under shoulders and flat on ground. Hold for 4–8 breaths or more.

POINTERS: Feel a two-way stretch between head and heels. Keep your weight lifted out of your shoulders, so that you feel light on your hands. Breathing is even and deep on inhalation and exhalation into your abdomen to avoid tensing the abdomen while holding the position.

B VASISTHASANA—THE INCLINED PLANK: From Plank Pose position A, keeping body as a straight line from feet through shoulders and head, open your right arm to point upwards, with body opening to face the right side, so weight rests between your left hand and the outside of your left foot with feet remaining flexed, legs together. Feel two-way stretch between feet and crown of head, while also feeling two-way stretch between opposite hands. Body is held in one straight line from head to heels. Look down towards your left hand. Hold for 3–5 breaths. Repeat to other side.

C For a simple option, start on all fours and open hips and shoulders to face the right with right arm extending upwards and extend the right leg diagonally down to the ground with foot lightly flexed. Look down towards left hand. Hold in this position for 3–5 breaths then repeat to other side.

A.

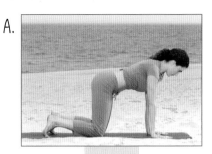

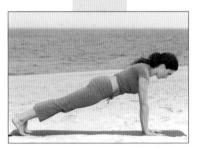

B.

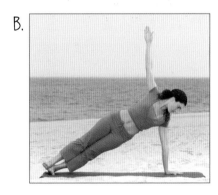

C.

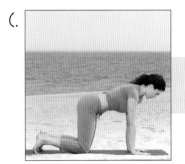

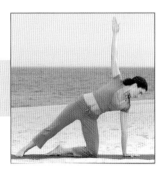

Push-up Series

STARTING POSITION: start in the Plank Pose (page 85).

A Carry out 8 push-ups, keeping your torso and legs extended as you lower your body as close to the ground as you can with elbows opened out to sides, and return to the plank pose 8 times. For an easier option, place knees on the ground with knees further back than your hips. Cross your ankles one on top of the other. From this position, carry out the push-ups. Then move into position B, keeping knees on ground.

B **INDIAN PUSH-UP POSITION:** From plank pose, lower your body to position suspended just above the ground, with elbows bent and held in at your sides. Hold for 3–5 breaths. Then move into position C.

C **COBRA:** From position B, lower body to ground, releasing toes so feet lie flat on ground. Then inhaling, raise chest and head upwards into Cobra position with elbows bent in at sides, hands supporting position on the ground with shoulders pressed down so neck is long. Hold for 3–5 breaths. Then move on to position D.

D **DOG STRETCH:** Raise hips into Dog Stretch position. Hold for 2–5 breaths.

Return to the Plank Pose to repeat the entire series from A to D. Repeat the series 3 times or more if desired.

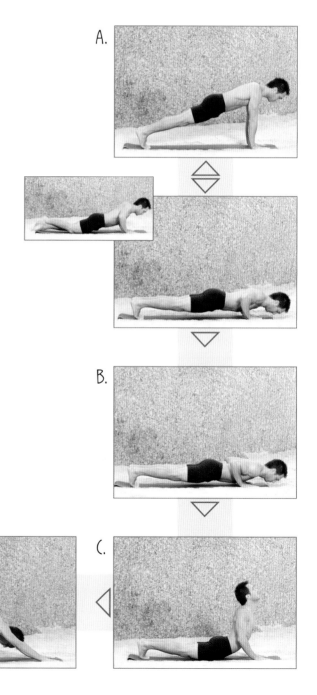

A.

B.

C.

D.

CHANDRASANA
Crescent Moon

A Start on all fours with toes pointed out behind you.

B Bring right leg forward between hands, placing sole of foot on ground. Lean hips forward to feel stretch across front of left hip. Check that right heel is under right knee so that there is a right angle at the right knee.

C Place right hand on right knee. Hold for 3–5 breaths.

Repeat to other side.

A.

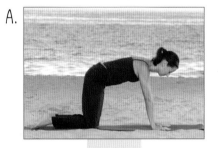

B.

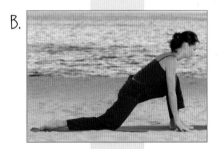

C.

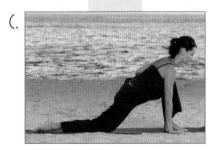

USTRASANA
The Camel

STARTING POSITION: Start sitting up on knees with legs slightly apart, hands at sides.

A DYNAMIC VERSION: From starting position, exhale and lean backwards maintaining straight line between knees and shoulders. Inhale recovering to upright, keeping hands at sides throughout. Repeat 8 times or more.

B Reach back to take hold of your right heel, with right hand, turning head to look down towards right foot. Left hand reaches to point vertically upwards. Hold for 3 breaths. Repeat to other side. If you cannot reach your heel, place right hand at back of right upper leg.

C USTRASANA: Keeping hips squarely facing front and in line over knees, bend backwards to take hold of both heels, arching spine, keeping hips forward in line over knees, with head following line of arch into back bend. Hold for 5 breaths. To recover, roll to one side via position B without the arm extending upward, simply hanging arms at sides, then curl body forwards over bent legs as you sit back toward your heels, then uncurl spine and sit up to starting position.

D Dynamic version with upper body circles: Start sitting up on knees with knees slightly apart, arms at sides. Inhaling, reach right arm sideways and up overhead to reach over into side bend to the left. Exhaling continue circling arm and torso to hang forwards, centred over legs, while slightly sitting hips back towards heels as spine relaxes forwards. Inhaling, continue the circle with left arm raising up to reach over in side bend to right side. Finally, exhale as return to starting position. Repeat 3 times in each direction.

A.

Inhale

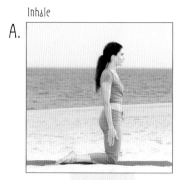

Exhale

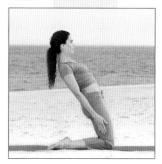

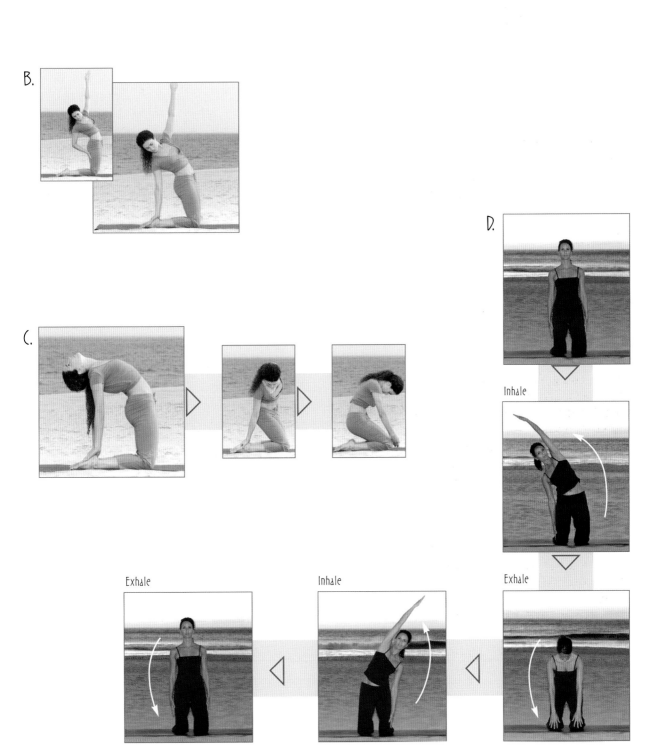

B.

C.

D.

Inhale

Exhale

Inhale

Exhale

TRANSITION TO STANDING

Spinal Rolling to Standing Position

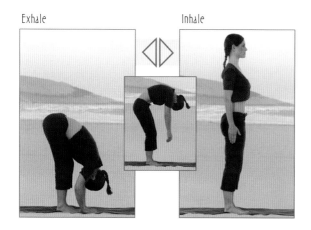

Exhale

Inhale

STARTING POSITION: Start on all fours with toes curled under. Feet are hip distance apart and parallel. Walk hands in towards feet, shifting weight onto feet with legs slightly bent, raise hips so that spine is relaxed and hanging forward over legs. Arms and head hang towards the ground.

Inhaling, uncurl spine to upright, straightening legs when upright and keeping feet well grounded throughout. Head comes up last.

Exhaling, curl down head first to position hanging forward over legs, knees bend slightly as you curl down. Dynamic version: Move from upright to forward bend 2 or 3 times to end in upright standing position.

Dynamic Frog Squat

A Start in a squat with knees bent and opened out to the sides, standing on the balls of your feet with heels off the ground touching. Fingers rest on the ground in front of your legs, with arms extended. Apply lock set # 2 (p. 53) and hold throughout.

B Inhale and raise hips as high as you can, extending your legs. Keep fingers on the ground with arms extending. Heels remain together. Head naturally moves towards legs in standing forward bend position.

Exhaling, lower to A. Repeat 8 times. Then rest for 4 breaths. Repeat all 2–4 times. This exercise tones the thighs and legs.

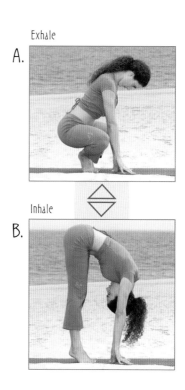

Exhale

A.

Inhale

B.

TADASANA
The Mountain Pose

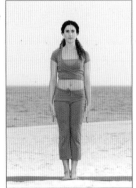

Exhale

A Stand with feet together. Knees are pulled up into thighs with legs pressed together. Arms and hands reach down at sides, with shoulders and chest open. Arms can either be touching legs or held slightly away. Spine is long. Head and eyes look straight out in front of you. Hold for 3–5 breaths, breathing into chest with lower abdomen slightly contracted (navel toward spine), so spine feels extended.

POINTERS: Weight is over 3 points of each foot, under big and little toe metatarsals and heels so you are well grounded through your feet. Shoulders are open and sternum (chest bone) is lifted slightly to allow the chest to be positioned slightly ahead of the abdomen. Feel sides of body equally lengthened, while grounded from waist down through feet and uplifted from waist up through neck and head. Hold chin parallel to the ground, or very slightly lowered towards the chest.

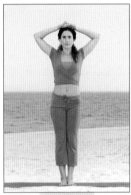

Inhale

B DYNAMIC RISES: Start in Tadasana position A. Place hands with fingers interlocked, on top of head, elbows open, palms facing up. Inhale, rising up onto your toes while extending arms and pushing hands upward, raising head to look up at hands. Exhale, returning to starting position with hands on head, head looking forward and feet flat. Repeat 8 times.

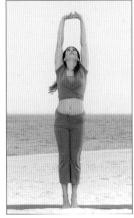

(**DYNAMIC SIDE BENDS:** Start in Tadasana with hands on head as for dynamic rises above. Inhaling, raise arms to push hands upwards. Head remains looking forward. Exhaling bend over to the right. Inhaling return to upright centre position with arms reaching upward. Exhaling bend over to the left. Inhaling return to centre again with arms raised. Feet flat on ground throughout.

Repeat 8 times in total (4 side bends each side alternately).

D **OPTIONAL COUNTERPOSTURE:** Clasp hands behind back palm to palm, extending arms upward behind you. Hold for 3 breaths, inflating chest on inhalation.

Exhale   Inhale   Exhale

C.
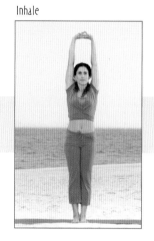 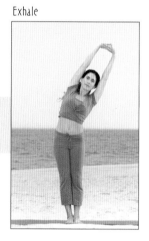

D.
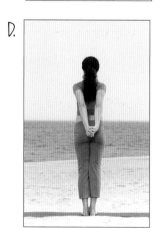

Dynamic Standing Side Bends

Stand with legs apart, arms parallel and reaching vertically upward alongside head, remaining extended throughout. Bend knees slightly with feet slightly turned out so position is comfortable. Keep your navel pressed in towards your spine throughout so lower back is stabilised.

A Bend upper body from side to side, breathing as feels natural, taking care not to strain by moving too fast. Repeat 8–12 times.

B Relax forward with head and hands hanging down towards the ground.

A.
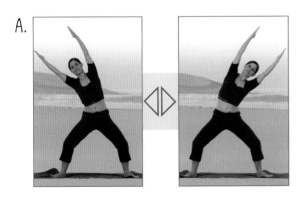

B.
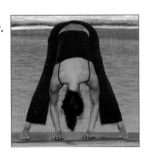

UTKATASANA
The Squat

A.
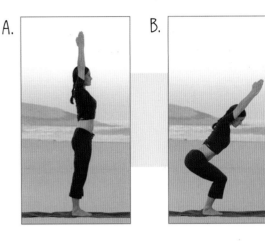
B.

A Start in Tadasana, then raise arms to parallel position reaching vertically upward alongside your head with chest slightly inflated as arms reach upward. Keep space between shoulders and ears. Part your heels slightly.

B On exhalation, bend knees as far as you can, keeping spine extending in two directions, hips reaching out behind you and arms reaching diagonally upward. Heels remain on ground with feet well grounded throughout. Head and neck remain in line with your spine, with back of neck extended and eyes looking diagonally down to the ground, ears alongside arms.
Hold for 3–5 breaths.

TO RECOVER: Reverse path taken into posture.

UTTANASANA
Standing Forward Stretch

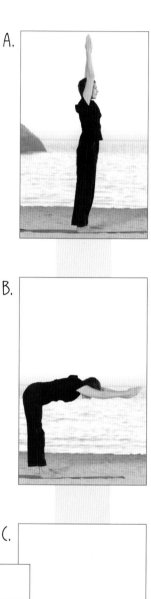

A.

A Start in Tadasana position A (p. 91). Inhaling, extend arms vertically upward alongside head.

B Exhaling, bend forward from your hips, keeping legs and spine extended, with legs pressed together for stability and knees pulled up into thighs throughout. Head remains in line with spine with arms alongside ears. Keep spine extended for as long as possible into the forward bend, rounding your spine at the very last stage to bring head toward legs.

B.

C Wrap hands around outsides of leg at a level that you can reach, such as calves, or ankles. Hold elbows in to sides of legs and keep bent to allow your arms to assist you in moving deeper into the forward bend. Ease abdomen toward thighs.

POINTERS: Feel tailbone reaching upward, with hips positioned over heels, weight slightly forward over balls of feet, so backs of legs feel long and extended. Feet are flat on the ground. Hold for 5 breaths.

Two options to recover: (i) The simple version is to bend knees and uncurl spine to upright starting position, bringing head up last with arms hanging relaxed as you uncurl to standing position. (ii) Reverse path taken into Uttanasana, starting by reaching your arms out ahead of you to position alongside head while extending your spine from tailbone through neck and head. Then recover to upright. Return to position with arms extended upward, then lower arms to sides into Tadasana starting position.

C.

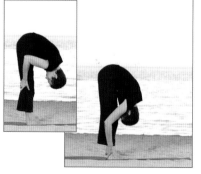

TRIKONASANA
The Triangle Pose

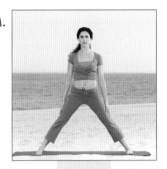

STARTING POSITION: With legs opened out to sides, a comfortable distance (just over a metre) apart, with feet parallel. Heels are in line with each other (you can line them up to the back of your yoga mat). Torso faces squarely to the front.

A Turn right foot and leg to point out to right side. Turn left foot slightly in, aiming for a 45 degree angle with toes pointing towards the right. Raise arms and hands to reach out to sides, at shoulder height, turning palms to face the front. Reach arms and torso to the right then bend sideways to the right to place your right hand on your right lower leg or ankle or on the ground behind your right foot; wherever you can reach. Left arm reaches upward. Feel two-way stretch between arms. Eyes look up to raised hand or, if your neck is uncomfortable, look out in front of you. To stabilise the position, feel spine well extended, knees pulled up into thighs so legs are well extended, and heels and feet firmly rooted into the ground with weight shared evenly between both legs. Hold for 3–5 breaths. To recover, reverse path taken into the position. Repeat to other side.

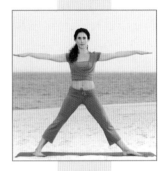

B With arm reaching over to extended side stretch: Start as for position A. When bending to the right, with left arm raised, reach extended left arm to point overhead to the right, maintaining straight line from left hand to hip in side bend, with torso more or less parallel to the ground. When bending to the left, right arm reaches overhead.

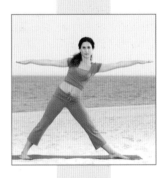

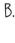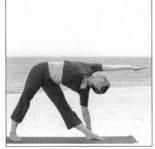

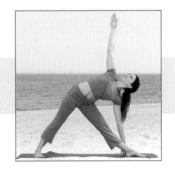

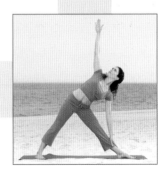

C Start in Trikonasana position A or B. When bending to the right, turn your hips and shoulders to face squarely over right leg in forward bend with hands on ground on either side of your right foot. If your flexibility does not allow you to reach the ground over two extended legs, then slightly bend your right leg. Keep spine long with head reaching forwards. Hold for a breath or two, feeling stretch to back of right leg.

D PARIVRITTA TRIKONASANA—THE REVOLVING TRIANGLE: Keeping legs in position C, inhale to open right arm to point vertically upward so torso twists to face the opposite side to Trikonasana, with two-way stretch between arms. Look up towards right hand or, if neck feels strain, look out in front of you. Hold for 3–5 breaths. To recover, reverse path taken into position.

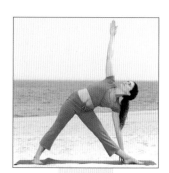

C.

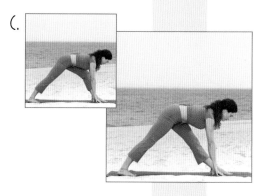

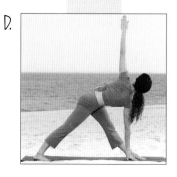

D.

VIRABHADRASANA 1
Warrior Pose 1

STARTING POSITION: start in Tadasana and open legs out to sides, a comfortable distance (just over a metre) apart, with feet parallel. Heels are in line with each other (you can line them up to the back of your yoga mat).

A Place hands on waist. Turn right foot and leg to point to right side. Turn left foot slightly in, aiming for a 45 degree angle with toes pointing towards the right.

B Bend right leg and turn hips and shoulders to face the right as squarely as possible. Weight is evenly distributed between both legs and feet. If you can, widen the position of your legs, working towards bringing your right thigh parallel to the ground with right knee in line over right heel. Right foot and knee point straight out in front of you. Eyes look forward.

C Raise arms and hands to reach upwards, fingers interlocked, palms facing upwards.

D Open arms to parallel position alongside head reaching vertically upward. Hold for 3–5 breaths. To recover, reverse path taken into position. Repeat to other side.

POINTERS: While holding position C and D, lift your chest slightly to allow arms to reach upward more easily. Feel your body stretched out in two directions—up through raised arms, and down through legs and feet with heels on the ground. Find steadiness by extending your spine and arms while centring your weight between both feet.

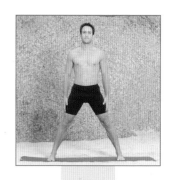

A.

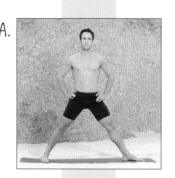

B.

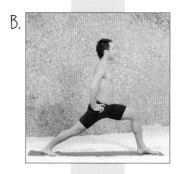

D.

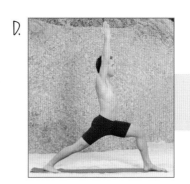

C.

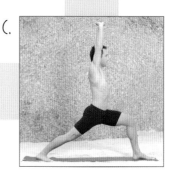

VIRABHADRASANA 2
Warrior Pose 2

A Start in Virabhadrasana 1 (p. 97) position with legs a comfortable distance apart.

B Keeping one leg bent and one leg extended, open hips and shoulders to face the front while opening arms out to sides in an 'archer' position. When right leg is bent, right arm extends out to right side at shoulder height, with palm facing forward. Left arm is bent with elbow pointing out to left side at shoulder height in line with right arm, with left palm facing in to your left shoulder. Fingers of both hands curled in to palms with thumbs extended to point upwards.
Look towards your right thumb, feeling a two-way stretch between both arms and feeling grounded through your legs with weight shared evenly between both legs. Spine is centred and long, breath expands chest on inhalation with chest and shoulders facing squarely to the front.

Hold for 3–5 breaths. Repeat to other side.

A.
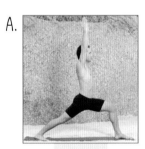

B.
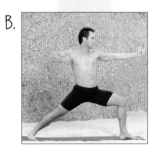

VIRABHADRASANA 3
Warrior Pose 3

A Move into Virabhadrasana 1 (p. 97) to the right, with legs a comfortable distance apart and arms on hips.

B Shift weight forward over bent right leg. Lower upper body to position more or less parallel to the ground, bringing abdomen towards right thigh, with arms reaching forward alongside head. Eyes look down toward the ground with spine extending. At the same time, raise extended left leg with foot pointing out behind you, aiming for straight line from head to toe. Feel two-way stretch between arms reaching forward and left leg reaching back.
Either hold in position B or C for 3–5 breaths.

C If you can, straighten your supporting leg, pulling knee up into thigh to stabilise the right leg and hold in this position.

To RECOVER: Bend supporting leg to return to Warrior Pose 1 with arms raised for one deep breath.
Then repeat balance to other side.

A.
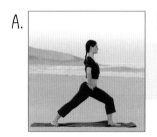

B.
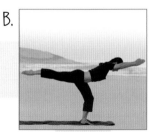

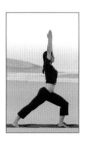

C.
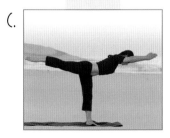

Dynamic Windmill Versions

STARTING POSITION: Stand with legs a comfortable distance apart and extended, with knees pulled up into thighs and feet slightly turned out to the sides.

A Inhaling, reach arms sideways and up to touch overhead. Exhaling, keeping hands touching with arms extended, reach down to touch right foot with fingertips. Inhaling return to upright centred position with arms reaching upward and repeat to left. Repeat 4–8 times each side alternately.

B Start with legs a comfortable distance apart, with knees slightly bent, feet parallel. Extend arms out to sides at shoulder height. Lean forward over legs to touch right hand to left foot, looking up to left hand with arms extending in opposite directions. Keeping torso more or less parallel to the ground, twist torso to other side, touching left hand to right foot. Repeat 8–16 times, with a swinging motion from side-to-side, keeping spine long with head reaching forward throughout. Then hang forward between legs with arms on or hanging towards the ground and hold for a deep breath or few.

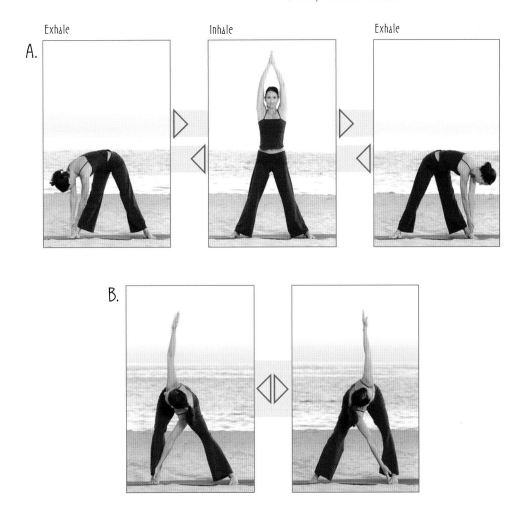

Counterpostures for Assymetrical Standing Postures

STARTING POSITION: Stand with legs open a comfortable distance (just over a metre) apart, with feet parallel. Bend forward from hips to hang over your extended legs.

ARM OPTIONS:

A Fold arms with arms hanging towards the ground.

B Relax arms toward the ground or to rest on the ground.

C Interlock thumbs behind back and raise extended arms up behind you as high as you can while hanging in forward bend over legs. For this version, before recovering, release hands and lower arms to hang before uncurling to standing position.

Hold for 3–8 breaths.

TO RECOVER: Bend knees then uncurl your spine to upright standing position, with head coming up last.

NOTE: If you have high blood pressure, only bend halfway down, perhaps placing your hands against a wall for support, with your head remaining above the level of your heart.

A.
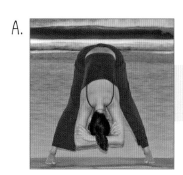

B.
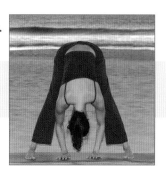

C.
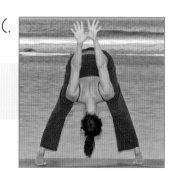

VRKSASANA
The Tree

STARTING POSITION: Start in Tadasana, position A (p. 91) with heels together or slightly parted. With the help of your right hand, raise your right foot to place the sole against the inside of your left leg, with right heel positioned as close in to your groin as possible. Open your right thigh and knee to point to the right side.

Place hands in prayer pose in front of your chest, with palms together, elbows opened out to sides. Eyes look out in front of you, finding a point of focus. Hold for 3–5 breaths.

POINTERS: Feel supporting leg stable with left foot grounded and knee pulled up into thigh. Feel spine extended. Remember balance is a state of mind. Will yourself to balance.

TO RECOVER: Return to Tadasana starting position. Repeat to other side.

NATARAJASANA
The Dancer

Start in Tadasana. Bend right leg to take hold of your right foot or ankle with your right hand, behind your hips. Keep your knees as close together as possible, so you feel a stretch across your right thigh. Raise your left arm to point vertically upward with hips and shoulders facing squarely to the front. Head and eyes look out front. This is a simple version of Natarajasana.

Hold for 3–5 breaths. Repeat to other side.

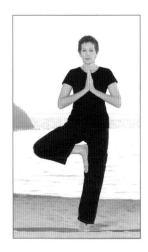

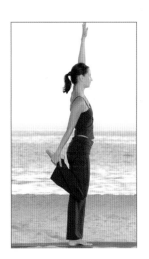

A Smooth Programme

This chapter consists of three sessions for slimming and toning three body areas (waistline, upper body and lower body). In addition, there is a short Yoga session for stretching and centring the body after a walk, run or other sporting or aerobic activity. There is also a short session for use when menstruating or to relieve premenstrual tension.

6. Yoga Sessions

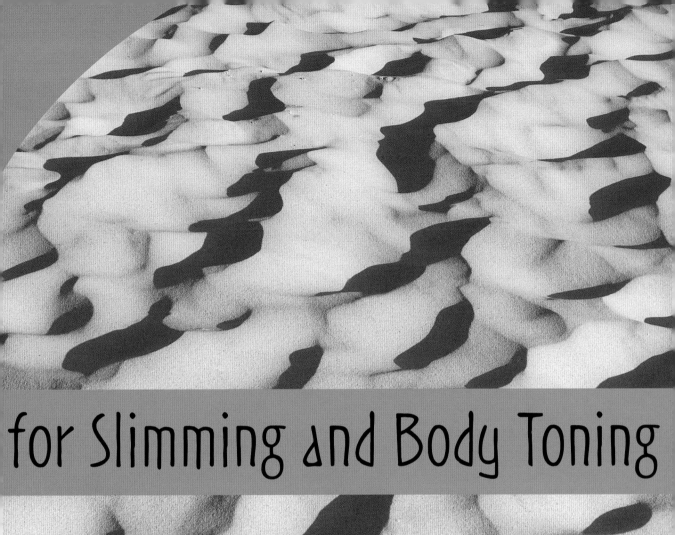

for Slimming and Body Toning

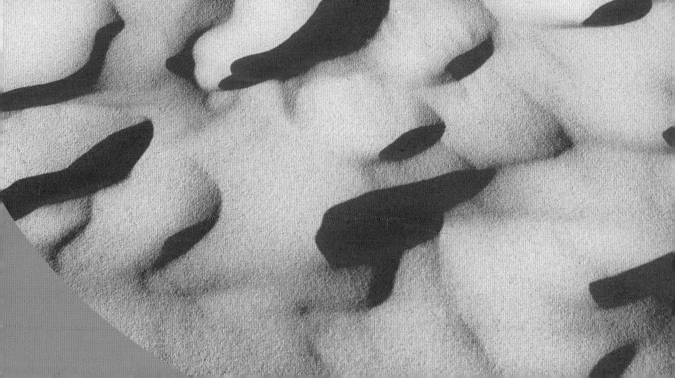

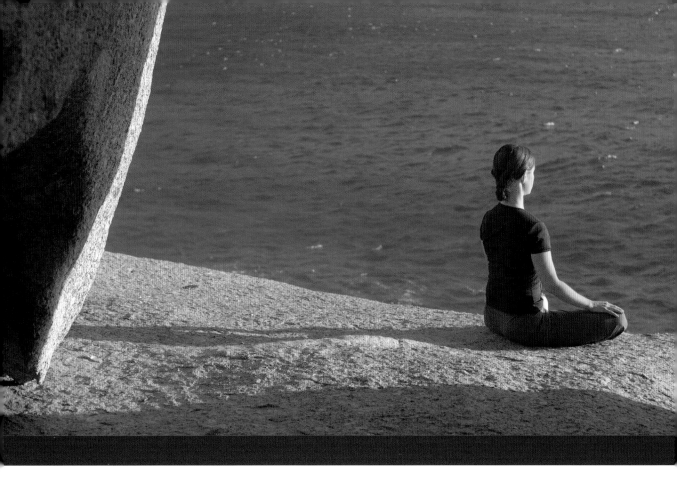

GENERAL NOTES

WHEN TO PRACTISE

• Find a time of day that works for you and practise consistently. Regular routine allows your body to accustom itself to the practice.

• Some prefer the early morning to prepare body and mind for the day. Others prefer the evening when the body is more flexible. An evening session is also an opportunity to unwind and centre. The two hours around sunset is recommended for evening sessions.

• In hot months of the year, avoid practising physical postures at the hottest time of day, although meditation is fine at this hour.

• Avoid practising straight after spending time outdoors in the hot sun.

• Never practise directly after eating. Wait half to one hour after a light meal and two to three hours after a heavy meal. The stomach should be empty.

• Empty your bladder and bowels if possible before practising.

• If you are menstruating, use the session designed for this time (see p. 110). Yoga flow #1 (p. 142) can also be used. These sessions can help relieve premenstrual tension.

WHERE TO PRACTISE

• Wherever there is an even, flat, firm surface, indoors or outdoors—in a garden or on the beach.

• A clean environment.

• Enough space for you to extend your arms and legs without obstruction, with space around you to move into and out of postures freely.

• The environment should be conducive to enjoyable practice with relative silence and a comfortable ambient temperature. An indoor area should be well ventilated. Practise outdoors only in moderate weather conditions: it should not be windy and neither too hot nor too cold, although you can wear extra layers of clothes. Find a place where you are least likely to be disturbed, although distraction can be used as opportunity to practise steady balance of mind and body.

HOW TO PRACTISE

How often: Maximum of 6 days a week, with at least one rest day.

How long: It is important to exercise for at least 30 minutes, but preferably an hour, daily. This is as essential as getting enough rest and eating regularly. Add 10–20 minutes meditation some time during the day. (You can start with five minutes a day and increase as you grow used to it.)

What to wear: Comfortable clothes that allow freedom of movement; preferably bare feet. Remove jewellery, watch and spectacles if possible.

What you will need:
- An exercise mat, preferably non-slip for better grip and stability in postures.
- Perhaps a cushion for meditation.
- Optional: A blanket if you wish to cover yourself while relaxing in Savasana at the end of the session.

CHOOSING SESSIONS

There are short sessions of about 10–15 minutes, as well as longer ones of 40–60 minutes. Below are a few ideas to help you design a programme.
General guidelines:
- Practise each of the 40–60 minute sessions at least once a week.
- You can choose to focus on a particular body area more often, as long as you still practise the other sessions at least once a week.
- The shorter sessions are recommended as specified.
- If you want a short session because you only have 5 or 10 minutes, use one or more of the sequences described in chapter 7, repeating at least one sequence four or five times. (The sequences in chapter 8 can also be included at the start or end of the 40–60 minute sessions for additional exercise).

SHORT SESSIONS
- 10 minute session before and/or after a run, walk, swim or other aerobic activity.
- 15 minute session when menstruating or to relieve premenstrual tension.
- Yoga flow posture sequences in chapter 7.

THREE SESSIONS FOR SLIMMING AND TONING DIFFERENT BODY REGIONS

Sessions generally take between 40–60 minutes. Allow extra time when you are doing them for the first time. Alternatively, do half the session until you are familiar with it and add extra postures over time until you are doing the full session within an hour. Always end with some time in Savasana (p. 54). Once familiar, sessions will progress more swiftly and smoothly.

All sessions include some focus on toning the thyroid gland to improve metabolism, which promotes healthy body weight. Each session focuses on specific body areas:
- Session 1: waistline—abdomen, lower back and sides of torso.
- Session 2: upper body—chest, upper back, shoulders and arms.
- Session 3: lower body—hips, buttocks and legs.

PROGRAMME IDEAS

Select a programme option that works best for you. In addition to any of these programmes, make time each day for 5–20 minutes of silent meditation, either at the end of a Yoga session, or first thing in the morning, or last thing at night before going to bed.

THE SESSIONS

Posture instructions: Full posture instructions are given in chapter 5. Each posture listed in this chapter is cross-referenced to a page number in chapter 5. Feel free to hold postures for longer than the suggested time.

Posture simplifications: These are specified in chapter 5 to assist you in achieving postures, and to ensure that there are posture versions available for different levels of ability. Always hold a simpler version of a posture rather than pushing yourself to achieve a posture for which you are not quite ready. Be assured that you will gain benefits from postures even at the very simplest level of execution. Over time, this is also a way to assess your progress as you find yourself able

Option 1

Day 1: session 1.
Day 2: preferred aerobic option (walk/ jog/ swim/ Yoga sequences), followed by the Short Session on page 108.
Day 3: session 2.
Day 4: aerobic option as for day 2.
Day 4: session 3.
Day 5: aerobic option.
Day 6: choose any of the 3 one-hour Yoga sessions for practice.
Day 7: rest.

Option 2

For 6 days per week do one of the 40–60 minute sessions, in chronological order and repeat. Add a 20-minute aerobic session 2 or 3 times per week (walk or jog outdoors, or swim; alternatively repeat the sequences in chapter 7). It is not necessary to do the aerobic session at the same time of day as your Yoga practice. Rest on day 7.

Option 3
based on a 5-day cycle

Day 1: session 1.
Day 2: session 2.
Day 3: session 3.
Day 4: aerobic session, followed by the short Yoga session on page 108.
Day 5: rest; perhaps do some Yoga sequence repetitions (see chapter 7) for 5–10 minutes.
Start 5-day cycle again.

to move into postures more easily. There are also options for more advanced practitioners. Leave these out if you are a beginner or if you try the posture and feel strain.

Posture selection and combination: There are many postures that benefit the body regions covered in this chapter, and many ways to combine postures. This book does not claim to cover all postures for toning respective body regions. Rather, the intention is to offer a selection of beneficial postures and combinations, presented as easy-to-follow sessions.

Leaving out postures: If you struggle to execute a particular posture, simply leave it out for now, trying it again when you are more Yogically 'fit'. Where possible, use simple versions of a posture rather than leave it out altogether. In the case of injury, consult your doctor and only do postures that do not strain the injured area.

Breathing while holding postures: Breathing is always through the nose unless otherwise specified. Breathe deeply and evenly on inhale and exhale. Breathing is used as a way to mark time while holding postures. It also encourages you to release unnecessary tension while holding postures.

Eyes are open while practising, unless otherwise specified.

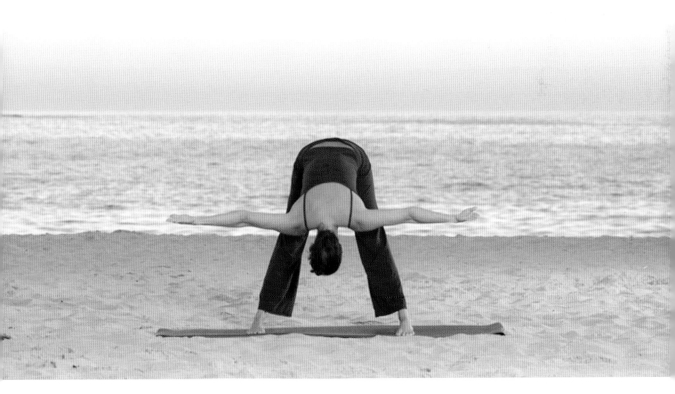

SHORT SESSIONS

10 MINUTE SESSION POST AEROBIC ACTIVITY (RUN, WALK, SWIM OR OTHER SPORT)

This session is for stretching, balancing, and centring the body. It can be used as a warm-up or a cool-down, or as a quick Yoga session option when you have little time. Gradually you will get to know this session so well that you can use it anywhere, anytime.

OPTIONAL Use a wall, table or chair-back for support.

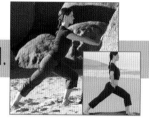 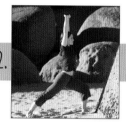 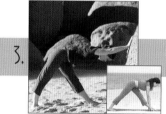 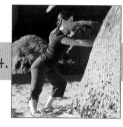

1. Virabhadrasana 1 (p. 97). With hands on waist or placed on support, press back heel into ground to feel calf stretch as well as stretch to front of left hip.
Hold for 2 or 3 deep breaths.

2. Hold the Warrior 1 (p. 97) position with arms raised, palms up with fingers interlocked. Hold for 3–5 breaths.

3. Parsva Uttanasana. From position 2, bend forward over front leg, straightening it as much as you can. Place hands next to front foot. Feel stretch to back of calf. Hold for 3 breaths. Repeat 1–3 with other leg.

4. Face front with feet parallel, legs apart. Lean forward, placing hands on support. Bend one leg at a time, feeling stretch to inner thigh. Hold for 2 breaths each side. Repeat.

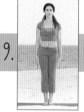 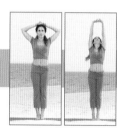 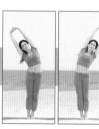 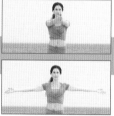

9. Tadasana (p. 91–92). Position A for one breath. Then use dynamic versions B and C with 8 rises and 8 side bends.

10. Arm swing. Standing in Tadasana (p. 91), swing arms open and closed a few times at shoulder height or just below.

5.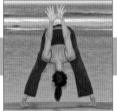

Counterposture. Hang forward over parted and extended legs. Bend legs slightly if necessary. Extend and raise arms behind you, thumbs interlocked. Hold for 5 breaths.

6.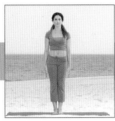

Tadasana (p. 91). Hold position A for 3 breaths.

7.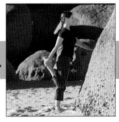

Natarajasana as thigh stretch (p. 101). Hold for 3 breaths each side, feeling stretch to your thigh. Optional: rest hands on support.

8.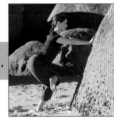

Cross an ankle over the opposite thigh. Raised leg has knee opened out to side. Bend supporting leg as if sitting on a chair. Hands rest on support or on legs. Feel stretch to outer side of hip of raised leg. Hold for 2 or 3 breaths each side.

11.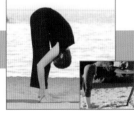

Uttanasana (p. 94). Hold for 3–5 breaths in forward bend over extended legs, with hands holding legs or resting on support. To recover, bend knees to uncurl spine, raising arms to reach upwards. Repeat 3 times.

12.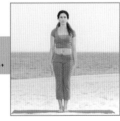

Return to Tadasana position A for one deep breath.

13.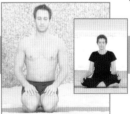

Meditation (p. 48). Sit in Vajrasana or with crossed legs for a few minutes of meditation.

15–20 MINUTE SESSION FOR WHEN MENSTRUATING OR TO RELIEVE PREMENSTRUAL TENSION

It is not advisable do a strenuous Yoga session while menstruating, especially not inverted postures or the bandha (energy locks). This session will help keep up your Yoga practice while menstruating, in an appropriate and gentle manner. Because this is a relatively short session, you can use the rest of the time for meditating.

5.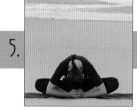

Baddha Konasana (The Butterfly) version C (p. 75) with hands holding feet. Hold for 5–8 breaths.

6.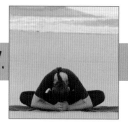

Upavista Konasana (The Straddle) (p. 76). Forward bend for 3 breaths. Side bends for 3 breaths each side. Then return to forward bend for 5 breaths.

7.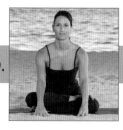

Baddha Konasana (The Butterfly) (p. 75), version C. Hold for 3 breaths.

8.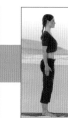

Crossed leg forward stretch (p. 78). Hold for 3–5 breaths. Repeat to other side.

12.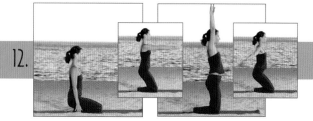

Rises sitting on knees—with arm circles: Inhaling, rise up to sit up on your knees while extended arms mark a half circle forward and up. Exhaling, sit back down on your heels as arms complete the circle, reaching back and down again. Repeat 2–4 times. Exercises 11 and 12 help balance the flow of subtle energies called Prana and Apana in the body, in support of healthy menstrual flow.

13.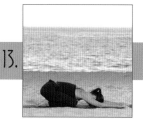

Supta Vajrasana (The Child Pose) (p. 82). With knees slightly parted, arms at sides. Hold for 5 breaths.

14.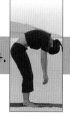

Spinal rolling to standing position (p. 90). Roll up and down spine 2 or 3 times, to end in standing position.

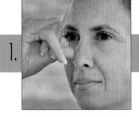 **1.** Nadhi Sodhana (p. 49): 8 rounds

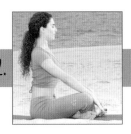 **2.** Full Yogic Breath (p. 50): 2 breaths

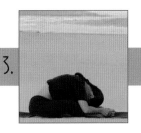 **3.** Simple Butterfly version (p. 75): Bending forward with hands holding feet, elbows opened out to sides and reaching down. Hold for 8 breaths.

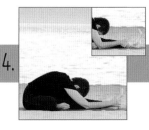 **4.** Janu Sirsasana (head to knee pose) (p. 70): First circle foot and ankle of extended leg a few times in each direction, hold for 5 breaths in forward bend each side.

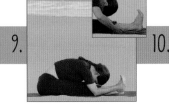 **9.** Pascimottanasana (Sitting Forward Bend) (p. 71). Hold in full forward bend for 5–8 breaths.

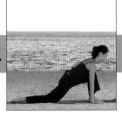 **10.** Chandrasana (Crescent Moon) (p. 87). Hold for 3–5 breaths each side.

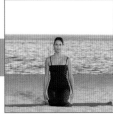 **11.** Rises sitting on knees. Sit on heels with legs folded under. Arms at sides. Inhaling, rise up on your knees, raise your arms to extend out to sides at shoulder height, palms facing down. Exhaling, return to starting position. Repeat 4–6 times.

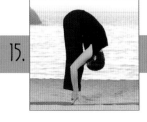 **15.** Uttanasana (standing forward stretch) (p. 94). Hold in forward stretch for 5 breaths. To recover, bend your knees and uncurl your spine, rolling up to a standing position with head coming up last.

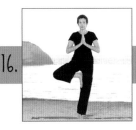 **16.** Vrksasana (The Tree) (p. 101). Balance for 5 breaths each side. To end, stand with legs together and arms at sides for a deep breath.

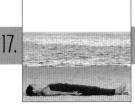 **17.** Savasana (The Corpse Pose) (p. 54). Roll down to sit, then lie on your back in Savasana. Rest for a few minutes.

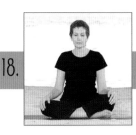 **18.** Meditation (p. 48). Sit in a comfortable cross-legged position, perhaps on a cushion.

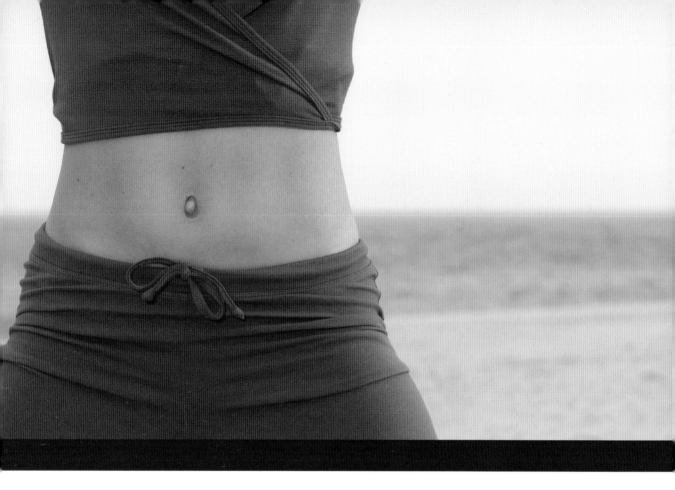

40—60 MINUTE SESSIONS FOR SLIMMING AND TONING DIFFERENT BODY REGIONS

WAISTLINE
ABDOMEN, LOWER BACK AND SIDES OF TORSO

Physical The waistline is the area surrounding the core of the body, a three-dimensional area between pelvis and diaphragm. The diaphragm is the sheet of muscle dividing the chest cavity from the abdominal cavity. In this core are the internal organs and muscles of the abdomen, as well as the lumbar vertebrae of the spine.

This area can powerfully generate energy from the core of our being as fuel for mind and body. It finds its grounding down through the hips, legs and feet. It finds its upliftment and interactive outlet through the upper body, including chest, arms, neck and head.

For slimming and body toning, Yoga postures offer a massage action to the internal organs, toning the organs, stimulating circulation of blood and lymph more freely to and from all body tissues, and improving digestion.

All body systems are improved as a result. Postures tone the muscles of this body region to a state of balance between tension and relaxation for optimal posture, core stability and lower back support. The breath of fire generates heat in the body for fat-burning. It also centres the body, tones the abdominal muscles and clears the mind.

Psychological association This area of the body is associated psychologically with the capacity for clarity, directness, and assertiveness in communication and action. It is also associated with expressing your 'gut feelings.' The tongue is connected to the throat at the upper end of the digestive tract that descends into the stomach, and from there further into the gut, which is associated with 'gut feelings'.

In the Yogic chakra system, the waistline includes the navel energy centre, called Svadhisthana chakra. It is associated with feeling centred and at home in your body. This is an important first step in a process of learning to love your body. In turn, this can motivate you to want to invest in your health.

The navel centre is a storehouse of vital and fiery energy for body and mind. It can also help control emotions. The way in which you deal with your emotions affects this body area. If you over-control your feelings you may hold in your abdominal muscles tightly. If you flow freely with your emotions, becoming overwhelmed by them and feeling helpless, your abdominal muscles may be slack. Some people eat for the feeling of fullness to dull painful emotions.

Toning the body in the way described in this session can generate a feeling of confidence in your ability to manage your emotions while continuing to feel centred in your body.

The waistline also includes the solar plexus energy centre called the Manipura chakra. This is the point of connection between 'gut feelings' of the lower body and the upper body, which houses your heart's passion and the seat of reason, your brain. Many people hold a knot of tension in this area, which may affect abdominal tone as a whole. It also affects breathing, which becomes shallow and restricted.

The ability to make and execute decisions is reflected here. Decision-making involves communication between gut-feelings, heart and head. When there is a conflict between reason, heart and gut feelings, it can be felt as a knot in the solar plexus area.

When feeling empowered the core area can give you feelings of worth, trust and comfort in your body and your sense of self. This supports your ability to make decisions with minimal stress and to be self-motivating.

All the more reason to tone this body region—for the slimness and shape you desire, but also for core stability and personal empowerment.

SESSION 1: SLIMMING AND TONING THE WAISTLINE. TIMING: 40–60 MINUTES

1.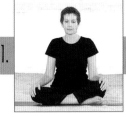

Ujjayi Breath (p. 48). 8 breaths sitting in a comfortable cross-legged position.

2.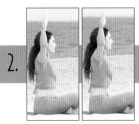

Agni Sara (Fire Breath) (p. 50). 20 to 100 Fire Breaths with arms raised. Optional: Afterwards apply lock set 2 then 3 (p. 53) for one held breath each, with hands on thighs.

3.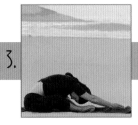

Simple Butterfly (p. 75) with Fire Breath. 20–40 fire breaths with thumbs interlocked, arms reaching forward. Then rest for 3 deep breaths relaxed forward over legs.

4.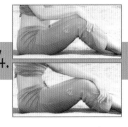

Lower back mobilising exercise (p. 68). 8–20 times or more. Then, remaining seated, apply lock set 2, then 3 (p. 53), holding for one breath each.

8.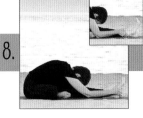

Janu Sirsasana (head to knee pose) (p. 70): Hold for 3–5 breaths each side in full forward stretch. Optional: with lock set 1 (p. 53).

9.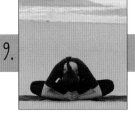

Baddha Konasana (The Butterfly) (p. 75) version C with hands holding feet. Hold for 5 breaths.

10.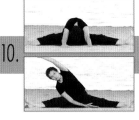

Upavista Konasana (The Straddle) (p, 76). Forward bend for 3 breaths. Side bend 2–3 breaths each side. Return to forward bend for 5 breaths.

11.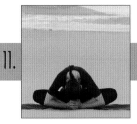

Baddha Konasana (The Butterfly). Return to Butterfly position C, holding feet. Hold for 3 breaths.

14.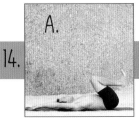

Dynamic leg raises (p. 58). Move between A and B 4 times.

15.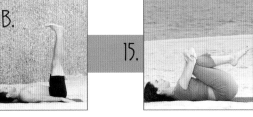

Apanasana (p. 55). Return to position A, hugging knees in over abdomen. Hold for 3 breaths.

16.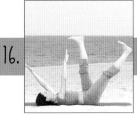

Leg walking (p. 59). Repeat version B 16 times.

5.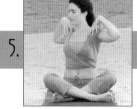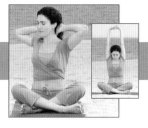

Upper body swing (p. 69). Do version A 8 times, B 8 times or more, then C with lock set 2, then 3, holding for one breath each.

6.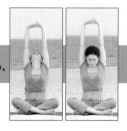

Neck stretch with arms raised, fingers interlocked. Inhale, looking up to hands, exhale looking down. Repeat 3 times.

7.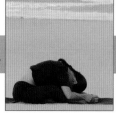

Simple Butterfly (p. 75). Version A with hands holding feet. Hold for 3–5 breaths. Optional: with lock set #1 (p. 53) applied.

12.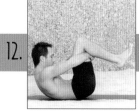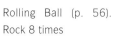

Rolling Ball (p. 56). Rock 8 times

13. 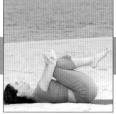 B. 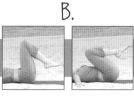 C.

Apanasana (p. 55). Hold A for 3 breaths. Then use dynamic version B 8 times and C 4 times in one direction, then the other.

17.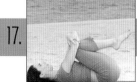

Return to Apanasana with knees hugged in over chest. Hold for 3 breaths.

18.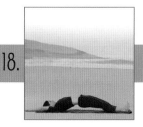

Body stretch with raised hips (p. 54). Sway hips side to side a few times, then return to lie flat on your back.

19.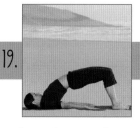

Setu Bandha Sarvangasana (The little bridge) (p. 60). Hold for 5–8 breaths. End on your back with knees hugged in over abdomen for 3 breaths.

20.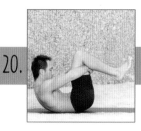

Rolling Ball (p. 56). Rock 4 or 5 times

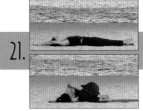

21. Dynamic body curls (p. 65). Curl twice to each side. End on your back with arms and legs extended in opposite directions.

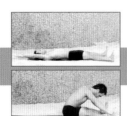
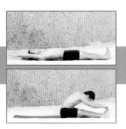

22. Dynamic sit-up (p. 64). Use version B, followed by C (4 times each).

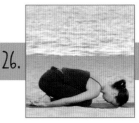

23. Pascimottanasana (Sitting Forward Bend) (p. 71). Hold in full forward bend for 5 breaths. Optional: with lock set #1 (p. 53).

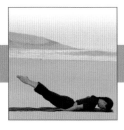

Hold in position C for 3–5 breaths.

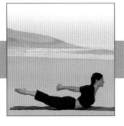

Hold in position D for 3–5 breaths.

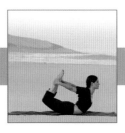

Optional: hold position E for 5 breaths.

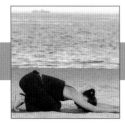

26. Supta Vajrasana (The Child's Pose) (p. 82), with arms at sides. Hold for 5 breaths.

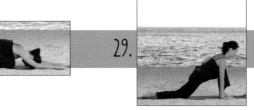

To end, rest for 3–5 breaths in the Child's Pose (p. 82), version with arms extended, elbows and forehead on ground.

29. Chandrasana (Crescent Moon) (p. 87). Hold for 3–5 breaths each side.

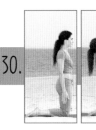

30. Ustrasana (Camel Pose) (p. 88). Use dynamic version A (8 times).

A. B.

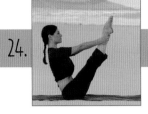 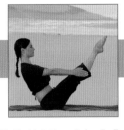

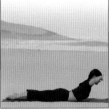

24. Navasana (The Boat) (p. 74). Hold A then B for 3–5 breaths. End sitting with knees hugged in to chest and hold for 2–3 breaths.

25. Preparatory series for Dhanurasana (The Bow) (p. 66). Hold in position B for 3–5 breaths.

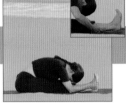

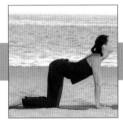 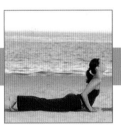

27. Pascimottanasana (sitting forward bend) (p. 71). Hold in full forward bend for 5 breaths. Optional: with lock set #1 (p. 53).

28. Bidalasana (Cat Stretch) (p. 83). Apply lock set #1 throughout. Version A (4 times).

Version B (4 times).

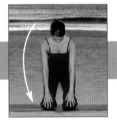

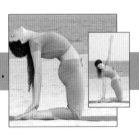

Dynamic version D (3 times) in each direction (p. 88).
Optional: Then rest in Child's Pose with arms at sides for a few breaths.

31. Ustrasana (Camel Pose) (p. 88). Held version: Hold either position B for 3 breaths each side, or C for 5 breaths.

32. 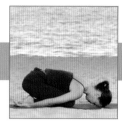 Supta Vajrasana (The Child Pose) (p. 82), with arms at sides. Hold for 5 breaths.

33. 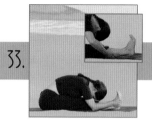 Pascimottanasana (sitting forward bend) (p. 71). Hold in full forward bend for 5 breaths. Optional: with lock set #1 (p. 53).

34. 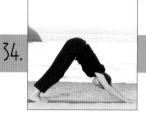 Adho Mukha Svanasana (Dog Stretch) (p. 84). Hold for 5 breaths.

35. 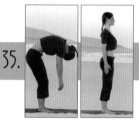 Spinal rolling to standing position (p. 90). Roll up and down spine 2 or 3 times, to end in standing position.

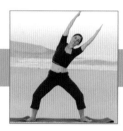 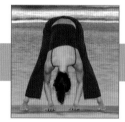 Then hang forward over bent legs for a few breaths, head and arms towards ground (p. 100).

38. 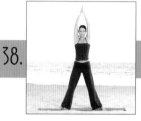 Dynamic Windmill (p. 99). Version A (4 times each side).

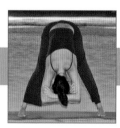 Then move into forward hang over extended legs (p. 100), arms folded.

41. 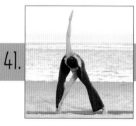 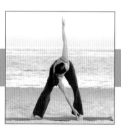 Dynamic Windmill (p. 99). Use version B 8–16 times.

Hang forward over bent legs, with arms relaxed to ground.

118

36.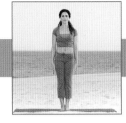

Tadasana (Mountain Pose) (p. 91–92). Hold position A for 3 breaths.

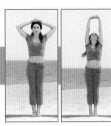

Dynamic version B 8 times.

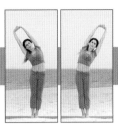

Dynamic version C with 8 side bends (4 to each side).

37.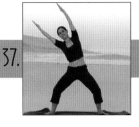

Dynamic side bends (p. 93). 8–12 side bends.

39.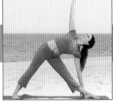

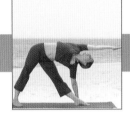

Trikonasana (The Triangle Pose) (p. 95). Hold position A then B for 3 breaths each.
Optional: Apply lock set #1 (p. 53) throughout.

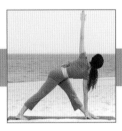

Trikonasana (The Triangle Pose) (p. 96). Hold position D for 3 breaths. Optional: Apply lock set #1 (p. 53).

40.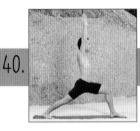

Virabhadrasana 1 (Warrior Pose) (p. 97). Hold for 5 breaths each side.

42.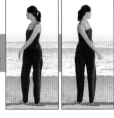

Standing twist swings. Feet hip distance apart and parallel, knees slightly bent. Twist upper body from side to side in a swinging motion. Swing about 8 times each side.

43.

Arm swings. Face front, legs extended. Swing arms open and closed 4–8 times.

44.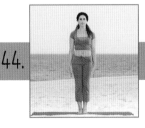

Tadasana (Mountain Pose) (p. 91). Hold position A for 3 breaths. Optional: With lock set #1 applied (p. 53).

45.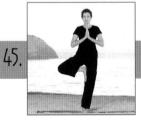

Vrksasana (Tree Pose) (p. 101). Balance for 5 breaths each side.
Then return to Tadasana for one deep breath.

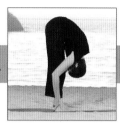

46. Uttanasana (Standing Forward Bend) (p. 94). Hold for 3–5 breaths. Optional: with lock set #1.

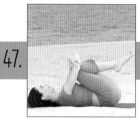

47. Apanasana (p. 55). Roll down spine to lie on your back with knees hugged in over abdomen for 3 breaths.

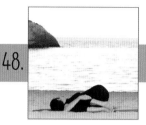

48. Jathara Parivartanasana (Spinal Twists) (p. 57). Hold A for 3–5 breaths each side. End in Apanasana, with knees hugged in over abdomen, for 2 breaths.

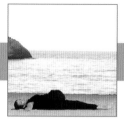

Hold B for 3–5 breaths each side.

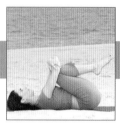

Hold in Apanasana, with knees hugged in over abdomen, for 3–5 breaths.

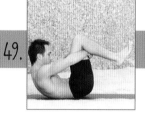

49. Rolling Ball (p. 56). Rock 4–6 times.

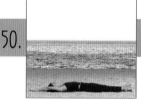

50. Lie on back, arms and legs extended. Inhale deeply and exhale, holding breath at end of exhale for as long as you can with lock set 3. Then take a deep breath.

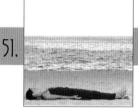

51. Savasana (The Corpse Pose) (p. 54). Rest for few minutes.

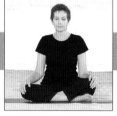

52. Ohm sound (p. 52) and meditation (p. 48). In sitting position, repeat ohm sound 3 times on long exhalations. Then move into meditation for a few minutes or more.

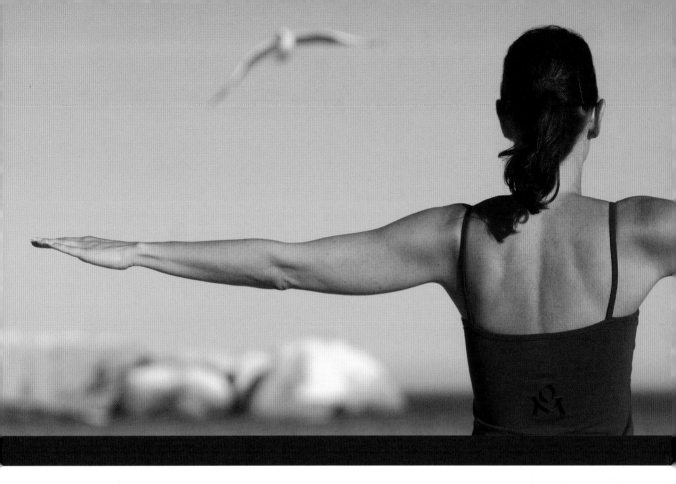

UPPER BODY
CHEST, UPPER BACK, NECK AND HEAD,
SHOULDERS AND ARMS

Physical This is the body region from the diaphragm up, including chest, shoulders and arms, neck and head. The chest houses the lungs and the heart, contained by the ribcage and supported from behind by the upper portion of the spine, both of which allow a certain amount of flexibility for breathing and body movement. The position of the chest in posture is related to the habitual positioning of the shoulders and arms, as well as how we hold our spine, neck and head. It is supported by an energised core of the body and stability in the hips, legs and feet.

This Yoga session is particularly effective for toning the thyroid gland in the neck area. This improves metabolic health, helping to stabilise body weight and energy levels. In addition, this session tones and shapes the arms and chest area, increases lung capacity through chest expansion, and generates a feeling of upliftment in body and mind. This upliftment helps you swiftly restore and maintain an optimistic state of mind through life's ups and downs as you move toward your goals.

Psychological association The psychological association of this body region relates to the four uppermost Yogic chakras or subtle energy centres. First there is the heart centre, known as the Anahata chakra. This is associated with feelings of love, appreciation and affection. The upper back can be viewed as the back door to the heart, where we may store defensive, reactionary feelings generated by lack of love or past hurt, and anger. The arms are the extension of this heart energy for giving and receiving in the world. Health involves receptiveness and softness at times, and the strength to say no and set a boundary at other times.

Breath, emotions and inspiration are also seated here. Inspiration has a way of uplifting the spirit and can fend off depression, while providing a sense of focus, purpose and enthusiasm. Added to this is feeling self-confident and self-assured; qualities that are more easily generated when this body region is toned.

The neck and head contain the three uppermost chakras. Together with the heart chakra they are associated with higher consciousness and awareness. Visuddha Chakra, at the throat, corresponds to the neck and jaw area. This area is associated with communication and the passage of energy between head and heart, between thinking and feeling. Confidence in speaking authentically and with authority has to do with the health of the throat area. The thyroid gland is housed in the throat, so the psychological association of this area with communication can influence the healthy functioning of the thyroid.

The brow energy centre, the Ajna chakra, sometimes referred to as the 'third eye', helps us balance the spiritual and the intellect. This energy centre is associated with rational, logical thinking.

The Ajna chakra plays a role in clearing, opening and illuminating the crown energy centre, the Sahasrara chakra, at the top of the head. This is associated with greater awareness. The feeling is that of deep inner peacefulness, perhaps even bliss, while feeling 'at one' with all aspects of oneself and with life and the universe.

SLIMMING AND TONING THE UPPER BODY

1.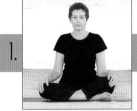

Ujjayi Breath (p. 48). 5 breaths.

2.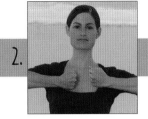

Brahmari (p. 51). Repeat 3 times using version A with chest tapping.

3.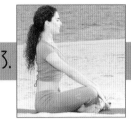

2 Full Yogic breaths (p. 50).

4.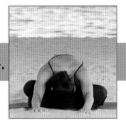

Hang torso and head forward, hands to ground. Restfully hold for 5 breaths.

5.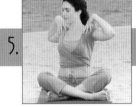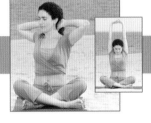

Upper body swing (p. 69). A and B (8 times each). Then do C with lock set 2, then 3 (p. 53), holding for one breath each.

6.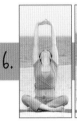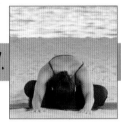

Neck stretch with arms raised, fingers interlocked. Inhale to look up to hands, exhale to look down. Repeat 8 times.

7.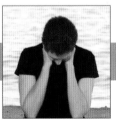

Hang torso and head forward, hands to ground. Restfully hold for 3 breaths.

8.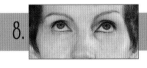

Eye exercises (p. 79). 3 circles in each direction. Optional: use all suggestions for eyes on p. 79. To end, rest eyes on ground diagonally down in front of you with soft, steady focus for 5 breaths.

9.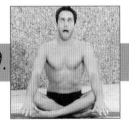

Simhasana (The Lion Breath) (p. 52). Hold for 3 breaths. Then relax your face and articulate the vowel sounds as a stretch for your mouth once or twice.

10.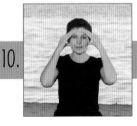

Face massage. Briefly massage your face and head including jaw and ears (to stimulate lymph circulation) and the back of your neck.

11.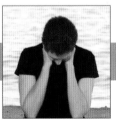

Neck stretches (p. 79). Forward for 3 breaths.

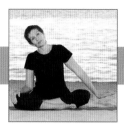

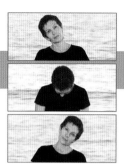

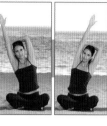

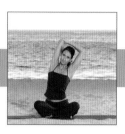

Stretch sides of neck, holding fo 2 breaths each side. Then do 2-4 neck rolls. End by returning to forward hang for 3 breaths.

12. Arm stretch series (p. 80). A through E on each side. Thereafter move on to positions F through I, holding for 2–5 breaths each.

13.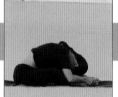

Simple Butterfly (p. 75). Version A with hands holding feet. Hold for 5 breaths.

14.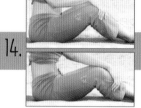

Lower back mobilising exercise (p. 68) 8–20 times. Then, still in sitting position, apply lock set 2 then 3 (p. 53), holding for one breath each.

15.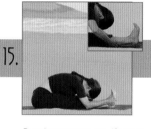

Pascimottanasana (Sitting Forward Bend) (p. 71). Hold in full forward bend for 5 breaths. Optional: with lock set #1 (p. 53).

16.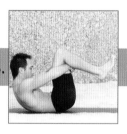

Rolling ball (p. 56). Rock 8 times.

20.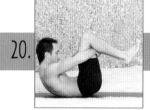

Rolling ball (p. 56). Rock 4 times.

21.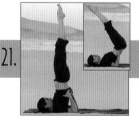

Supported Shoulder Stand (p. 61). Hold position A or B for 5 breaths.

22.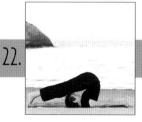

Optional: Halasana (The Plough) (p. 62). From the shoulderstand, move into Halasana. Apply lock set #1 (p. 53). Hold for 5 breaths.

23.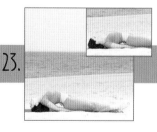

Matsyasana (The Fish) (p. 63). Hold position A or B for 5 breaths.

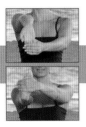
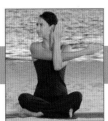
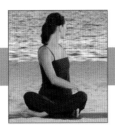
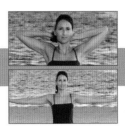
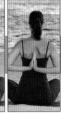
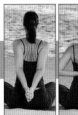

17.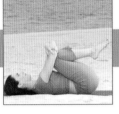

Apanasana (p. 55). Hold position A for 3 breaths.

18.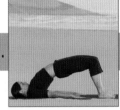

Dynamic leg raises (p. 58). Move between A and B 4–6 times.

19.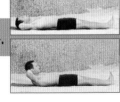

Setu Bandha Sarvangasana (The Little Bridge) (p. 60). Hold for 5–8 breaths. End lying on back with knees hugged in over abdomen for 1 or 2 breaths.

24.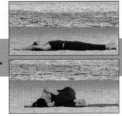

Dynamic partial sit-ups with extended legs (p. 64). Dynamic version A 8 times.

25.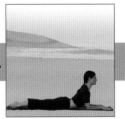

Dynamic body curls (p. 65). Curl twice to each side. End by lying on your back. Then flip over to lie on your front.

26.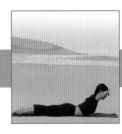

Preparatory series for Dhanurasana (The Bow) (p. 66). Hold position A for 3–5 breaths.

Hold position B for 3–5 breaths.

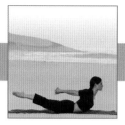

Hold position D for 3–5 breaths.

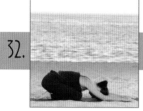

Optional: Hold position E for 5–8 breaths.

27.

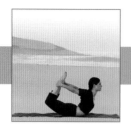

Supta Vajrasana (The Child's Pose) (p. 82). With arms at sides. Hold for 5 breaths.

28.

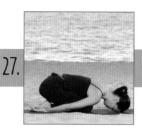

Optional: Urdhva Dhanurasana (The Full Bridge) (p. 60). Hold for 5 breaths. Then hold Apanasana A, hugging knees over abdomen for a few breaths.

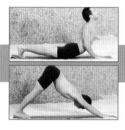

Inhale to C in cobra, then exhaling to D in dog stretch. Repeat series A–D 3 times.

32.

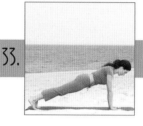

Supta Vajrasana (The Child's Pose) (p. 82). With arms extended and forehead, hands and elbows on the ground. Hold for 5 breaths.

33.

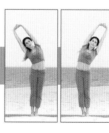

Plank series (p. 85). A and B or C. Hold for 5 breaths each.

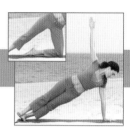

38.

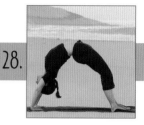

Tadasana (Mountain Pose) (p. 91–92). Hold position A for 3 breaths.

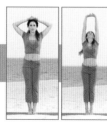

Dynamic version B with 8 rises.

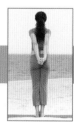

Dynamic version C with 8 side bends (4 each side).

Then use counterposture with arms extending behind you with hands clasped for one or two deep breaths.

29.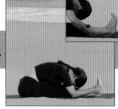

Pascimottanasana (Sitting Forward Bend) (p. 71). Hold in full forward bend for 5–8 breaths. Optional: Hold with lock set #1.

30.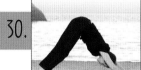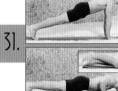

Adho Mukha Svanasana (Dog Stretch) (p. 84) for 5 breaths. Optional: Rest for 3–5 breaths in the Child Pose.

31.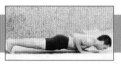

Push-up series (p. 86) A (8 push ups).

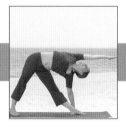

Then lower into Indian push-up pose B to hold for a breath or two.

34.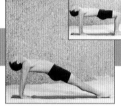

Half Bridge (p. 72). Hold in position D or simpler version A for 5 breaths.

35.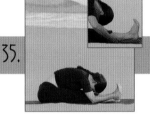

Pascimottanasana (Sitting Forward Bend) (p. 71). Hold in the full forward bend for 5 breaths with lock set #1.

36.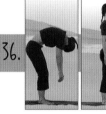

Spinal rolling to standing position (p. 90). Roll up and down spine 2 or 3 times, to end in standing position.

37.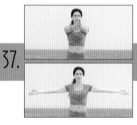

Arm swings open and closed a few times approximately at shoulder height.

39.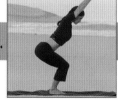

Utkatasana (The Squat) (p. 93). Hold for 3–5 breaths. Optional: with lock set #1.

40.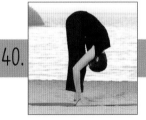

Uttanasana (Standing Forward Stretch) (p. 94). Hold in forward stretch for 5 breaths with lock set #1 applied.

41.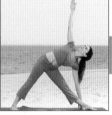

Trikonasana (The Triangle Pose) (p. 95). Hold position A then B for 3–5 breaths each.

42.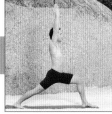

Virabhadrasana 1 (Warrior Pose) (p. 97). Hold for 5 breaths. Then move directly into Warrior 2 before repeating to other side.

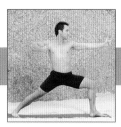

Warrior Pose 2 (p. 98). Hold for 3–5 breaths. Then repeat Warrior 1 and 2 to other side.

43.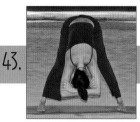

Hang forward over extended legs, feet parallel, legs a comfortable distance apart. Arms folded (p. 100). Hold with lock set #1 for 3–5 breaths.

47.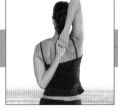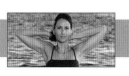

Gomukhasana arm position (p. 82). Hold for 3–5 breaths each side. Then hook fingers behind neck with elbows open and hold for 3 deep breaths.

48.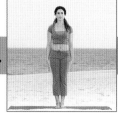

Tadasana (Mountain Pose) (p. 91). Hold position A for 3 breaths.

49.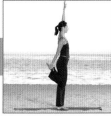

Natarajasana (The Dancer) (p. 101). Balance for 3–5 breaths each side.

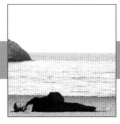

Hold B for 3–5 breaths each side.

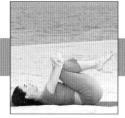

Hold in Apanasana, with knees hugged in over abdomen, for 3 breaths.

54.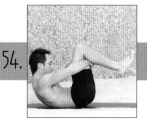

Rolling Ball (p. 56). Rock 5–8 times. End by sitting, then lying back down.

55.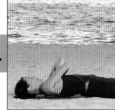

Self hug: Lying in relaxed position on your back, cross arms over chest to hold sides of ribcage under your armpits. Hold for few easy breaths feeling the sense of self-acceptance and self-love that this position offers.

44.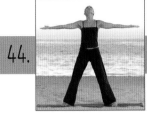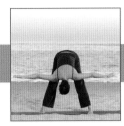

Forward and backward bend over parted legs. Inhale bending backward, exhale bending forward 8 times.

45.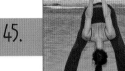

Hang forward over parted legs with arms behind you extending upwards, thumbs interlocked (p. 100). Hold with lock set #1 for 5 breaths.

46.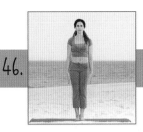

Tadasana (Mountain Pose) (p. 91). Hold position A for 1 deep breath.

50.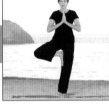

Vrksasana (The Tree) (p. 101). Balance for 3–5 breaths each side.

51.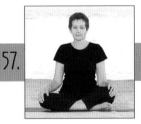

Tadasana (Mountain Pose) (p. 91). Hold position A for 1 deep breath.

52.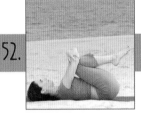

Apanasana (p. 55). Hold A for 3–5 breaths.

53.

Jathara Parivartanasana (Spinal Twists) (p. 57). Hold A for 3–5 breaths each side. End in Apanasana, with knees hugged in over abdomen, for 2 breaths.

56.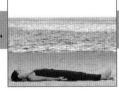

57.

Savasana (The Corpse Pose) (p. 54). First use Brahmari version B (p. 51) 3 times, humming on extended exhalation with lips closed. Feel the vibration throughout your body. Then rest for a few minutes in Savasana.

Ohm sound (p. 52) and meditation (p. 48). In sitting position, repeat ohm sound 3 times on long exhalations. Then move into meditation for a few minutes or more.

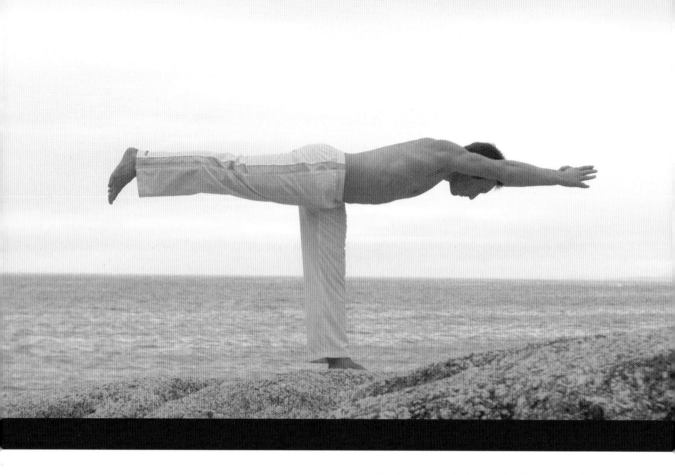

HIPS, BUTTOCKS AND LEGS

Physical This area originates in the pelvic region and extends down to the ground through legs and feet. The main functions are to ground the body and facilitate movement. Grounding serves as foundational support and stabilisation necessary for uprightness, for walking or other forms of locomotion.

Psychological association The pelvic region is home to the root or base energy centre, called Muladhara Chakra in Yogic philosophy. The legs and feet are extensions of the root energy centre. This area relates to basic survival instincts, sense of security and feeling grounded or rooted in the physical world. This can then serve as a foundation from which higher consciousness can arise.

FEELING EMPOWERED

The root chakra is an important power centre in the body. Energy is generated here for circulation through the body. For this reason, this body region reflects our relationship to feelings of power, control, independence and assertiveness. When out of balance, we can feel frustrated, insecure, fearful and unstable. The ability to stand up for ourselves in an empowered way is associated with the hips and legs. Expressions such as 'taking a stand' or 'standing on your own two feet' or 'standing up for yourself' indicate this association.

Particular Yoga postures in standing positions require you to pay attention to the position of your hips and the stability of your legs to help you find your balance. Pressing your navel in toward your spine in postures encourages stabilisation of the lower spine and hips. In your legs, stability involves finding the balance between muscular tension and relaxation so you can feel grounded through your feet. This helps you to feel powerful, while being able to move your upper body freely.

The root energy centre can also carry emotional baggage related to sexuality and the ability to let go, or the ability to assert yourself. Yoga practice can help you to put your two feet on the ground, stand up for yourself and move forward in life in meaningful ways, regardless of what has happened in the past.

SENSE OF DIRECTION IN LIFE

The legs and feet are associated with forward movement and sense of direction in life. Feeling grounded through hips, legs and feet can offer stability and clarity of direction to body and mind. The hips represent our inner formulation of direction through association with our creative reproductive centre. Any issues we may have in this area, such as weight accumulation, can relate to issues around creativity.

Walking your path is the means for grounding your creativity, dreams and inspirations in practical reality. Legs relate to our capacity to feel supported and empowered about walking on our life path in a direction we feel good about.

Legs and feet literally carry us forward in our direction of choice. They also help to facilitate our survival instincts, such as fleeing, fighting or freezing in situations of perceived danger. In light of this, when our legs are strong and function well for us, we can feel safer in the world.

For slimming and body toning, this session is particularly effective for promoting eliminative health, such as digestive and circulatory health. In so doing, it supports your body to eliminate excess fatty deposits and waste materials as effectively as possible. The session also tones this body region, balancing strength and flexibility to promote a desirable shapeliness in your hips, buttocks and legs.

The session can also support you in taking a stand for yourself and your life, and in walking your life path, in a way that feels grounded, stable and energised.

1.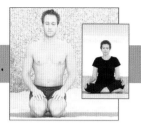

Ujjayi Breath (p. 48): 10 breaths sitting in Vajrasana with legs folded under, or sitting on heels with hands on thighs. Alternatively sit comfortably with crossed egs.

2.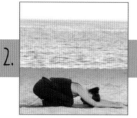

Supta Vajrasana (The Child's Pose) (p. 82): With arms extended and forehead, hands and elbows on the ground. Hold for 5 breaths.

3.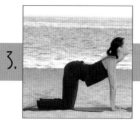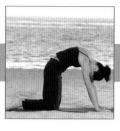

Bidalasana (Cat Stretch) (p. 83): Version A 5 times. Optional: with lock set #1 (p. 53).

8.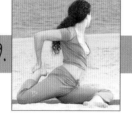

Baddha Konasana (The Butterfly) (p. 75): With hands holding feet. Hold for 5 breaths.

9.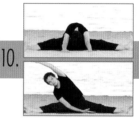

Version of Eka Pada Rajakapotasana (The Pigeon) (p. 77): Hold for 3–5 breaths each side, feeling stretch to the thigh of the leg that is behind you.

10.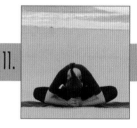

Upavista Konasana (The Straddle) (p. 76): Forward bend 3 breaths. Side bends 2–3 breaths each side. Then return to forward bend 5 breaths.

11.

Baddha Konasana (The Butterfly) (p. 75): Return to Butterfly position C holding feet. Hold for 3 breaths.

15.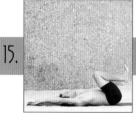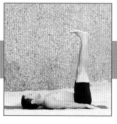

Dynamic leg raises (p. 58): Move between A and B 4 times.

16.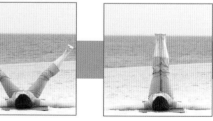

Leg walking (p. 59): A repeat 8 times then B repeat 16 times.

4.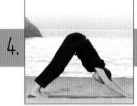

Adho Mukha Svanasana (Dog Stretch) (p. 84): Hold for 5 breaths in position A.

5.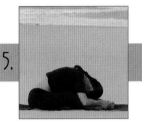

Simple Butterfly (p. 75): Take a few moments to massage your feet in this position, then hold feet and open elbows as you relax in forward bend for 3–5 breaths.

6.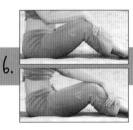

Lower back mobilising exercise (p. 68): 8–20 times or more. Then, remaining in sitting position, apply lock set 2 then 3 (p. 53), holding for one breath each.

7.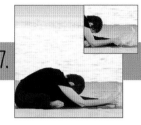

Janu Sirsasana (Head to knee pose) (p. 70): First circle foot and ankle a few times in each direction. Then move into forward bend and hold for 5 breaths with lock set 1 (p. 53). Repeat to other side.

12.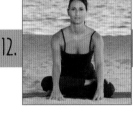

Crossed leg forward stretch (p. 78): Hold for 3–5 breaths each side.

13.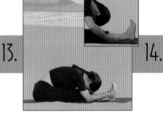

Pascimottanasana (Sitting Forward Bend) (p. 71): Hold in the full forward bend for 5–8 breaths. Optional: with lock set #1 (p. 53).

14.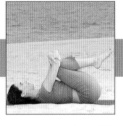

Apanasana (p. 55): Hold position A for 3 breaths

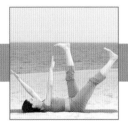

17.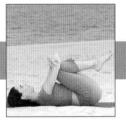

Return again to Apanasana with knees hugged in over chest. Hold for 3–5 breaths.

18.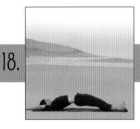

Body stretch with hip sway (p. 54): Sway hips a few times from side to side.

19.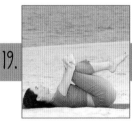

Apanasana (p. 55): Hold position A for 3–5 breaths.

20.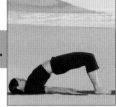

Setu Bandha Sarvangasana (The Little Bridge) (p. 60): Hold for 5–8 breaths. End lying on your back with knees hugged in over abdomen for 3 breaths.

21.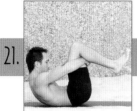

Rolling Ball (p. 56): Rock 8 times.

22.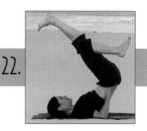

Supported shoulder stand (p. 61): Move into position A then follow instructions for B, kicking your buttocks with your heels alternately, 16 times or more.

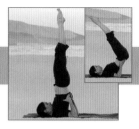

Hold in position A or B for 5 breaths.

27.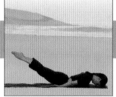

Preparatory series for Dhanurasana (The Bow) (p. 66): Hold position C for 5 breaths.

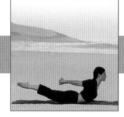

Hold position D for 5 breaths. Then optional rest with head on hands for 8 breaths before moving on to swimming versions.

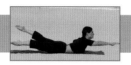

Swimming versions F (i) and (ii), alternately repeating 2 or 3 times each.

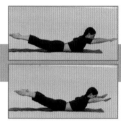

Dynamic version C (i) With one leg crossed over the other, pulse hips in small motion up and down 8 times. Repeat with other leg.

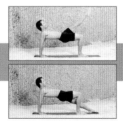

Dynamic version C (ii) raising and lowering one extended leg 4–8 times. Repeat with other leg.
Optional: Rest for a few breaths in sitting position.

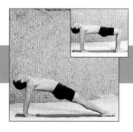

Hold position D or A for 3–8 breaths. For either option, head can hang backwards or if neck feels strained, keep head raised to look toward navel.

31.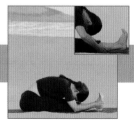

Pascimottanasana (sitting forward bend) (p. 71): Hold in the full forward bend for 5–8 breaths. Optional: with lock set #1 (p. 53).

23. 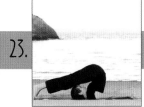 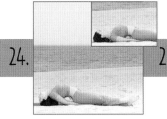 Optional: Halasana (The Plough) (p. 62): From the shoulderstand, move into Halasana position A. Apply lock set #1 (p. 53). Hold for 5 breaths.

24. 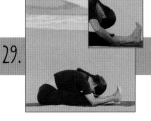 Matsyasana (The Fish) (p. 63): Hold position A or B for 3–5 breaths.

25. 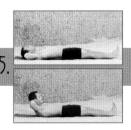 Dynamic partial sit-ups with extended legs (p. 64): Dynamic version A 8 times.

26. 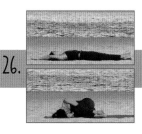 Dynamic body curls (p. 65): Stretch out body then curl to one side then the other alternately. End lying on your back.

28. 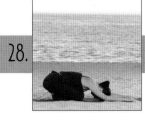 Supta Vajrasana (The Child's Pose) (p. 82): With arms extended, forehead, hands and elbows on the ground. Hold for 5 breaths.

29. 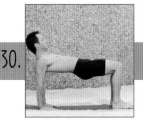 Pascimottanasana (Sitting Forward Bend) (p. 71): Hold in full forward bend for 5 breaths. Optional: with lock set #1 (p. 53).

30. 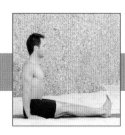 Half Bridge (p. 72): Dynamic version B 8 times.

32. 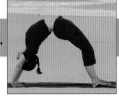 Optional: Urdhva Dhanurasana (The Full Bridge) (p. 60): Hold for 5–8 breaths. Move into Apanasana for 3–5 breaths, hugging knees in over abdomen, then return to position 31, then 33.

33. 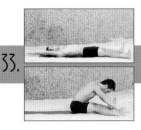 Dynamic sit-up versions (p. 64): B, 4 times.

33. 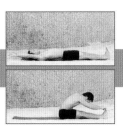 Dynamic sit-up version C (p. 64) 4 times.

34. 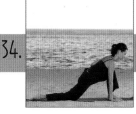 Chandrasana (Crescent Moon) (p. 87): Hold for 3–5 breaths each side.

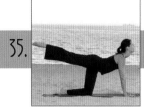 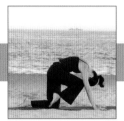 **35.** 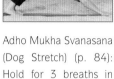 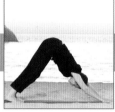 **36.**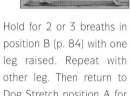

Bidalasana (Cat Stretch with leg extension) (p. 83): Use dynamic version C 4 times with one leg then the other.

Adho Mukha Svanasana (Dog Stretch) (p. 84): Hold for 3 breaths in position A.

Hold for 2 or 3 breaths in position B (p. 84) with one leg raised. Repeat with other leg. Then return to Dog Stretch position A for 2 or 3 breaths.

41. 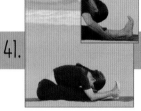 **42.** 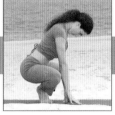 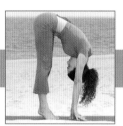 **43.**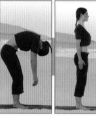

Pascimottanasana (Sitting Forward Bend) (p. 71): Hold in the full forward bend for 5 breaths. Optional: with lock set #1 (p. 53).

Frog squat (p. 90): 8 hip raises, 2–4 times in total, resting between rounds. Apply Lock set #2 (p. 53) throughout.

Spinal rolling to standing position (p. 90): Roll up and down spine 2 or 3 times, to end in standing position.

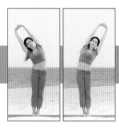 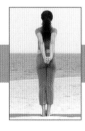 **48.** 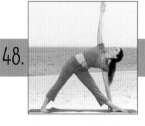 **49.**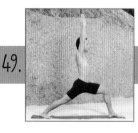

Dynamic version C (p. 92) with 8 side bends (4 side bends each side alternately).

Then use counterposture with arms extending behind you with hands clasped for one or two deep breaths.

Trikonasana (The Triangle Pose) (p. 95): Hold for 5 breaths in position A. Repeat to other side.

Virabhadrasana 1 (Warrior Pose) (p. 97): Hold for 5 breaths. Then move directly into Warrior 2 before repeating to other side.

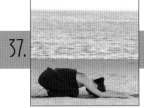 **37.**

Supta Vajrasana (The Child's Pose) with arms extended (p. 82). Hold for 3–5 breaths.

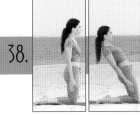 **38.**

Ustrasana (Camel Pose) (p. 88): Use dynamic version A 8–16 times, inhaling to upright, exhaling to backward tilt.

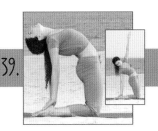 **39.**

Ustrasana (Camel Pose) (p. 88): Hold either position B for 3 breaths each side, or position C for 5 breaths.

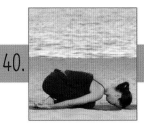 **40.**

Supta Vajrasana (The Child's Pose) (p. 82): With arms at sides. Hold for 5 breaths.

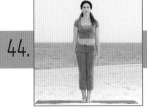 **44.**

Tadasana (Mountain Pose) (p. 91): Hold position A for 3 breaths.

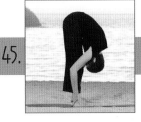 **45.**

Uttanasana (Standing Forward Stretch) (p. 94): Hold in forward stretch for 5 breaths.

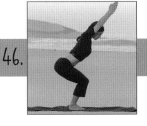 **46.**

Utkatasana (The Squat) (p. 93): Hold for 3–5 breaths. Optional: with lock set #1 (p. 53).

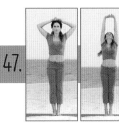 **47.**

Tadasana (Mountain Pose) (p. 91): Dynamic version B with 8 rises.

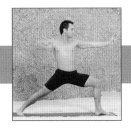 **50.**

Warrior Pose 2 (p. 98): Hold for 3–5 breaths. Then repeat Warrior 1 and 2 to other side.

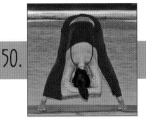 **51.**

Hang forward over extended legs (p. 100): Arms folded. Hold with lock set #1 (p. 53) for 3–5 breaths.

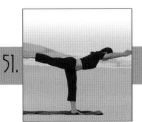 **52.**

Virabhadrasana 3 (Warrior Pose balance) (p. 98): Hold balance with supporting leg bent or straight, for 3–5 breaths each side.

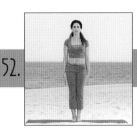

Tadasana (Mountain Pose) (p. 91): Hold position A for 3 breaths.

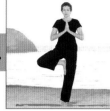

53. Vrksasana (The Tree) (p. 101): Balance for 3–5 breaths each side.

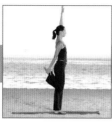

54. Natarajasana (The Dancer) (p. 101): Balance for 3–5 breaths each side.

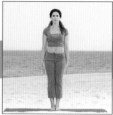

55. Return to Tadasana position A for 3 deep breaths.

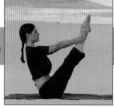

58. Navasana (The Boat versions) (p. 74): Hold position A for 3–5 breaths.

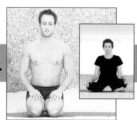

Optional: Hold position C (p. 74) for 3–5 breaths. To end, move into sitting position for a few breaths, hugging knees in to chest with head curled in to knees.

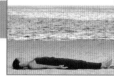

61. Savasana (The Corpse Pose) (p. 54): Rest for few minutes.

62. Meditation (p. 48): Meditate for a few minutes or more, sitting with legs folded under or cross-legged.

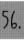 **56.**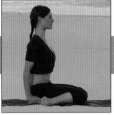

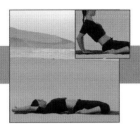

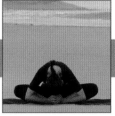 **57**

Optional: Supta Virasana (p. 78): Hold in position A, B or C for 3–5 breaths. You can sit on a cushion if you need to.

Baddha Konasana (The Butterfly) (p. 75): Version C with hands holding feet. Hold for 3–5 breaths.

59.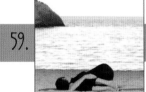

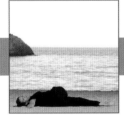

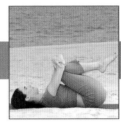

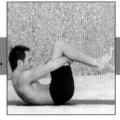 **60.**

Jathara Parivartanasana (Spinal Twists) (p. 57): Hold A for 3–5 breaths each side. End lying on back with knees hugged in over abdomen, for 2 breaths.

Hold B for 3–5 breaths each side.

Hold in Apanasana (p. 55), with knees hugged in over abdomen, for 3 breaths.

Rolling Ball (p. 56): Rock 6–8 times.

What is a Yoga Flow or Vinyasa?

Vinyasa (also known as vinyasa krama) refers to two or more Yoga postures strung together in sequence. In Sanskrit, 'Vi' means separating and 'nyasa' means placing or putting down. A characteristic feature of vinyasa is smooth, flowing transitions between postures, with movement coordinated with breath. For this reason, Vinyasa is translated here as a Yoga flow.

The Yoga flows in this book are easy to memorise. Once memorised and familiar, they become short Yoga session options for use as an energising start to your day if you do not have much time in the morning, or as a tool for relaxing, de-stressing or unwinding at the end of your day. They can be used as accompaniment to a Yoga session or as short sessions on their own.

When used repeatedly, Yoga flows can have an aerobic effect on the heart, especially if continued for at least 20 minutes. This offers a cardiovascular 'work-out' option through Yoga.

Yoga flows carried out slowly and meditatively have a calming, soothing effect on the nervous system. This offers a remedy for a modern, high-stress lifestyle, serving as an antidote to the fast-pace of the working world. Used in this way, Yoga flows can alleviate or prevent the accumulation of stress and tension.

Benefits of Yoga flows can be experienced on many levels:
» Improves blood circulation throughout the body, increasing oxygen supply to the body and brain.
» Increases stamina and strength
» Cultivates ease, flow and grace in movement by facilitating integration of all body parts in motion
» Improves co-ordination through the flow of one posture into the next where all body parts are invited to move harmoniously with each other.
» All Yoga flows support slimming and toning of the entire body and aid in achieving and maintaining ideal weight. Yoga posture flows:
» Promote healthy circulation of blood and lymph to and from body tissues in support of tissue nourishment and efficient waste removal.
» Provide a massage to internal organs in service of their healthy functioning. This is achieved by posture combinations that alternately stretch and compress body parts in relation to each other.
» Enhance lung capacity, promoting higher energy levels and mental clarity as the body and brain are oxygenated. This is achieved by co-ordination of breath with Yoga postures.
» Tone the endocrine system promoting healthy metabolism involved in stabilising our energy levels, burning fat and promoting immune system health.
» Have a natural energising effect. This can encourage us to follow through on our healthy lifestyle and move toward meaningful life goals.

GENERAL NOTES:
» *Flows are applied repetitively.*
» *For more of a 'work-out', use more repetitions.*
» *You can use more than one sequence in a session for a comprehensive 'work-out'. In this case, use one Yoga flow a few times before moving on to the next.*
» *Breathing is through your nose; is co-ordinated with movement; is deep and even on inhalation and exhalation.*
» *Moving slower builds strength and endurance. Moving faster develops agility and lightness. It is recommended to start slowly while familiarising yourself with positions to avoid injury through recklessness.*

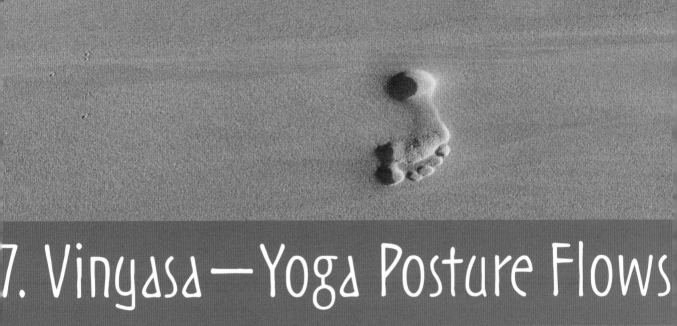

7. Vinyasa—Yoga Posture Flows

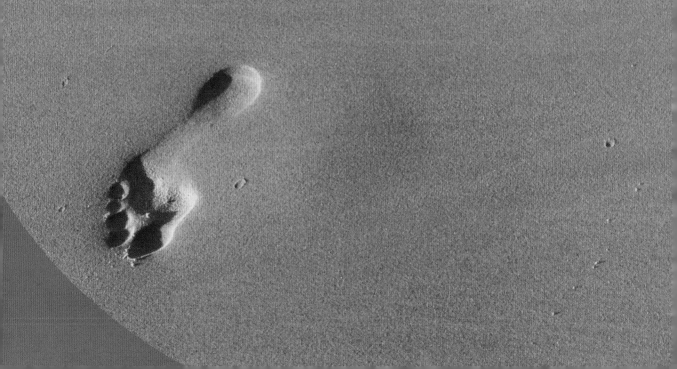

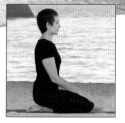

1.

START in Vajrasana, sitting with legs folded under, hands on thighs.

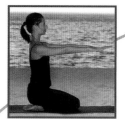

10. **Inhale:** Raise arms up to shoulder height in front of you, palms down. **Then exhale**: lowering arms to return to starting position on thighs in Vajrasana.

Repeat 3 times or more

Yoga Flow 1: Gentle, Calming, Soothing

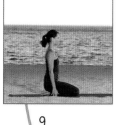

Exhale: Sit back down on your heels, arms fan out and down sideways.

9.

Inhale: Uncurl to sit up on your knees with arms raised alongside head.

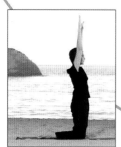

8.

Exhale: Child's Pose, arms along-side head on ground.

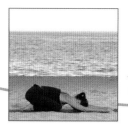

7.

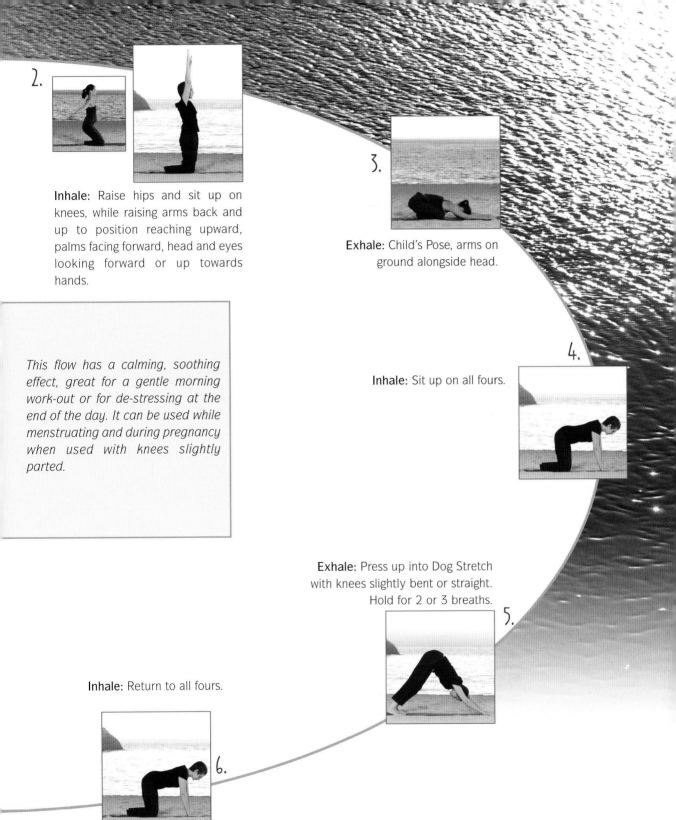

2.

Inhale: Raise hips and sit up on knees, while raising arms back and up to position reaching upward, palms facing forward, head and eyes looking forward or up towards hands.

3.

Exhale: Child's Pose, arms on ground alongside head.

This flow has a calming, soothing effect, great for a gentle morning work-out or for de-stressing at the end of the day. It can be used while menstruating and during pregnancy when used with knees slightly parted.

4.

Inhale: Sit up on all fours.

Exhale: Press up into Dog Stretch with knees slightly bent or straight. Hold for 2 or 3 breaths.

5.

Inhale: Return to all fours.

6.

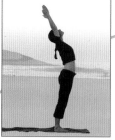

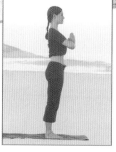

Start in Tadasana with hands in Prayer Pose.

1.

11. **Inhale:** Reach arms and torso forward and up to return to standing position with arms raised.
Then exhale: lowering arms to starting position in Prayer Pose.

Repeat 6 times or more

Yoga Flow 2: Sun Salutation

This Sun Salutation combines a variation of Yoga postures to limber, stretch, tone and strengthen your entire body. It is to be carried out in a smooth, flowing manner.

Exhale: Step left leg forward, placing left foot next to right, with knees bent then straightened as much as you can.

10.

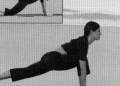

Inhale: Step right leg forwards, reaching spine and head forwards, placing right foot between hands with right knee bent at a right angle, knee over heel. Left leg remains extended or bends behind you with toes on the ground.

9.

Exhale: Raise hips into Dog Stretch.

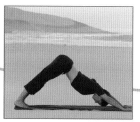

8.

2.

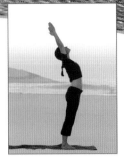

Inhale: Raise arms to reach up and slightly back as you bend your upper body backwards, with eyes looking up towards your hands.

3.

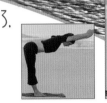

Exhale: Move into forward bend, placing hands on ground next to feet, bending knees if you need to.

4.

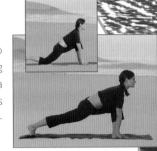

It can be used slowly as a gentle warm up or cool down to a Yoga session, or as a short session on its own. This Yoga flow can also be applied as a cardiovascular work-out if desired, with multiple repetitions of the same sequence. Or you can follow this Yoga flow with Yoga flow 3, for variation and a more comprehensive work-out.

Inhale: Step right leg out behind you to place toes on the ground with leg extended or bent. Left leg is bent at a right angle, knee over heel. Spine is long, reaching spine and head forwards.

Exhale: Step left leg back to join right leg in Chaturangasana.

5.

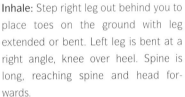

Hold breath: Lower body into Indian Push-Up position, with body suspended just off ground and elbows in at sides. Alternatively, use simpler option, lowering chest, knees and forehead to the ground in the Caterpillar position, with hips raised and elbows in at sides.

6.

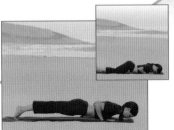

Inhale: Lower body to the ground and move into Cobra position, with chest, head and chin raised so looking upward. Elbows are in at sides and slightly bent.

7.

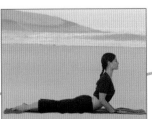

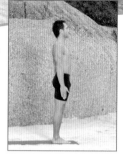

Start in Tadasana.

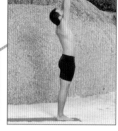

10. **Inhale:** Uncurl to standing position then raise arms sideways to reach upwards, looking up to hands.
Then exhale: lowering arms sideways and down to return to starting position in Tadasana.

Repeat 3–5 times or more

Yoga Flow 3: Sun Salutation

This is a more strenuous version of a Sun Salutation.

Exhale: Return to forward bend position, bringing head towards legs.

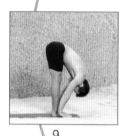

9.

Inhale: Jump feet forward between hands. Head and spine reach diagonally forward, legs are bent on landing from jump, then straighten as much as you can.

Exhale: Bend and straighten elbows as you move into the Downward-Facing Dog Stretch.
Hold for 3–5 breaths.

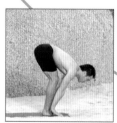

8.

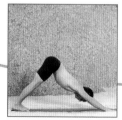

7.

2.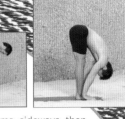

Inhale: Raise arms sideways and up to touch overhead with chin raised, eyes looking up to hands.

3.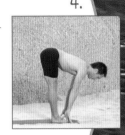

Exhale: Lower arms sideways then down as lower head then torso into forward bend with spine rounding till in forward bend with head tucked in towards legs. Hands on ground next to feet with legs straight or slightly bent.

4.

Inhale: Reach spine and head diagonally forward from hips.

It can be used as a dynamic warm-up to a Yoga session, or as a short Yoga session on its own. This Yoga flow can also be applied as a cardiovascular work-out if desired, with multiple repetitions of the same sequence. Or you can precede it with Yoga flow 2 for variation and a more comprehensive work-out.

5.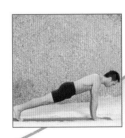

Exhale: Jump feet back into Chaturangasana.

Inhale: Bend and straighten elbows into Upward-Facing Dog Stretch, with toes curled under, hips and legs suspended above ground, spine and head reaching upward, and chin raised with eyes looking up.

6.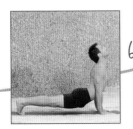

Do You Have a Medical Condition?

If you have a medical condition, it is advisable to seek medical or health specialist advice before embarking on a slimming and physical fitness program.

It is also advisable to consult with a health specialist especially through the initial transition period where side effects or detoxification symptoms could occur. This can help guide you into health with peace of mind, assisting your body to make the transition as easily as possible through any physical challenges that may accompany the initial stages of weight loss and getting fit. Examples may include nausea or headaches related to the body's cleansing process. If you do not experience these in extreme, then simply persevere with your new lifestyle program and the symptoms should pass in a week or so.

There are some conditions where doctor's consent and ongoing consultation is recommended especially during the initial month or three of a lifestyle change. These are as follows:

OBESITY: Exercise with caution, starting slowly and gently, perhaps practising a few postures at a time, gradually building up your practice. Be in regular consultation with a doctor to guide you through any issues that may arise while your body detoxifies and moves toward health.

HEART CONDITION: Avoid inverted positions where the head is held below the level of your heart, for example the Shoulder Stand and the Plough. If it is not a strain for you to do the Dog Stretch, hold for a minimal amount of time, such as a breath or two, perhaps resting in the Child's Pose then returning into the position again. You may need to avoid Vinyasa (chapter 7) so as not to strain your heart. If you feel you are straining during postures, relax for a few minutes in a rest pose or by relaxing your efforts, concentrating more on breathing and feeling grounded from your hips downward.

HIGH BLOOD PRESSURE: In this case avoid inverted postures, such as the Shoulder Stand and Plough position or hold for minimal amounts of time. For breathing, make your exhale longer than your inhale while practising Yoga postures. This can help regulate high blood pressure when practised consistently. The opposite is required for low blood pressure, where it is beneficial for inhalation to be longer than exhalation.

DIABETES: Healthy metabolic function involves metabolism of sugar towards energy production. Carrying out a health-oriented program as recommended in this book may result in your needing to adjust your insulin levels if you are insulin dependent. Be in regular consultation with your doctor about this.

PREGNANCY: Although this book is a great guideline for losing weight and getting back in shape after pregnancy, the programs in chapter 6 are not designed for use during pregnancy. However, there are some postures you can use.

During pregnancy, particularly the first two trimesters, you can use forward bending postures with legs parted to allow space for the abdomen. Sitting, kneeling and standing postures can be used without strain, perhaps holding for minimal amounts of time. You can rest between postures and repeat postures that are being held for short amounts of time.

The Child's Pose can be used as a rest posture with knees parted. Savasana can be adapted to resting on your side with a pillow between your knees. Simple back bends, such as the Camel Pose, are also fine, so long as you do not feel strain and obviously do not

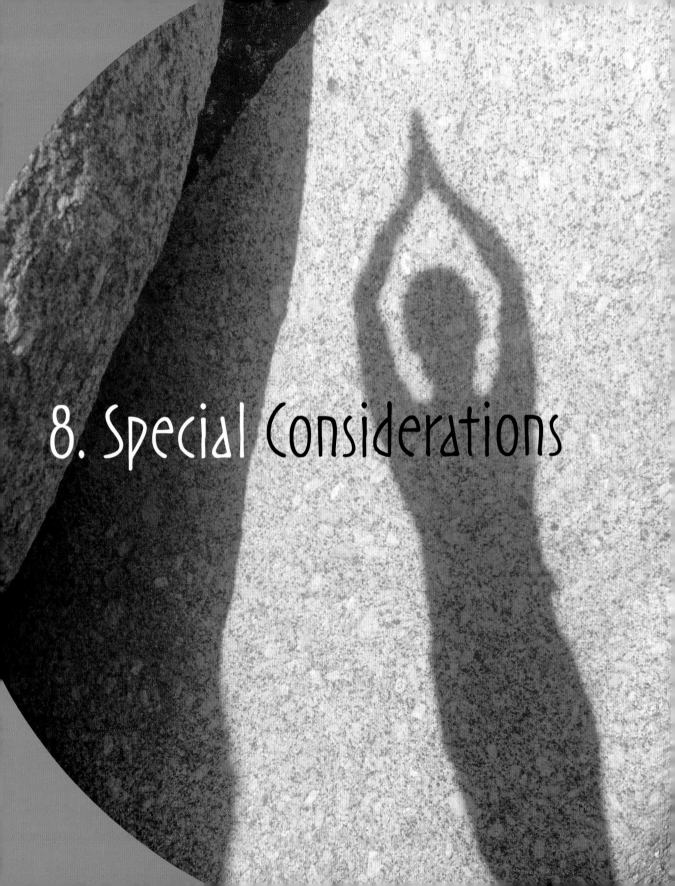

8. Special Considerations

use any postures that involve lying on your abdomen. As a general guideline, exercise in moderation during the first two trimesters of pregnancy. In the final trimester, avoid postures that are strenuous and stick to mild exercise. Also wait at least a month after giving birth before resuming an exercise practice.

POSTNATAL: Wait one month before resuming a mild exercise practice. By three months after childbirth you can safely resume all sessions and follow the programs offered in this book in support of resuming your ideal weight and shape. Directly after giving birth it is recommended to practise lock set #1 (p. 53) at regular intervals, perhaps using 10 repetitions at a time, holding for as long as you can each time you apply it while breathing naturally. You can even do this while carrying out your daily chores. This encourages return of muscle tone in the pelvic floor and lower abdominal area.

INJURY OR ILLNESS: For minor illness such as a common cold or flu, allow approximately one week after recovery before resuming your full exercise practice, starting slowly and gently during this time, perhaps only doing half of any of the sessions in chapter 6, or practising slow repetitions of the Yoga flows of chapter 7. Allow another week or more to build up your strength and stamina again. While you are ill, it may be possible and satisfying for you to do a simple stretch or two in a forward bend position, such as Pascimottanasana—sitting forward bend (p. 71), or Baddha Konasana—The Butterfly (p. 75), holding for a minute or few while breathing deeply and easily. Use your discretion about this. With illnesses where a doctor's consultation is required, consult with your doctor about when to begin exercising again and how strenuously. Practise with care, centring and toning the parts of the body you are able to work with.

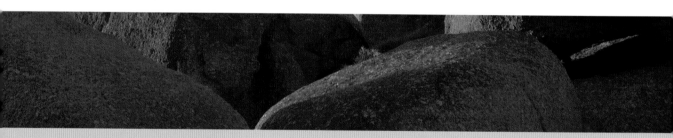

Acknowledgements

The author would like to thank Graeme Robinson for the magnificent photography, as well as for his patience and plenty of overtime that went into shooting and preparing the large number of pictures. Yoga models are Noa Belling, Claudia Gurwitz, Claudine Marich, Warren Munitz and Janetta Van Der Merwe. Thank you for giving your time and Yoga towards the creation of this book. For the Yoga clothing, thanks are due to Claudine Marich again for providing us with yoga wear from her range called 'Namaste Yoga and Exercise Wear'.

The author would like to thank all her Yoga teachers who have helped broaden and mould her Yoga awareness. Special mention goes to Ananda Kutir Yoga Ashrama in Cape Town, South Africa, where Noa completed her Yoga teacher training many years ago. Finally, the author wishes to thank Stephanie Mines, PhD, for passing on her wisdom on acupressure and its value in psychological health. Noa trained with Dr Mines in the TARA approach, which applies Jin Shin Acupressure for the resolution of shock and trauma in the body. Her influence can be seen in the psychology section on page 37 of this book alongside the Yogic 'Yoni'/'Sanmukhi' Mudra.

Index

Abdomen, 112–20
Addiction, 36
Adho mukha svanasana (Dog Stretch), 84, 118, 127, 133, 136, 143
Aerobic exercise, 26
Agni sara (fire breath), 50, 114
Apanasana (wind-relieving), 55, 114, 115, 120, 125, 128, 129, 133, 139
Arms
 cow-face posture, 82
 slimming and toning, 121
 stretches, 80, 81, 124
Arm stretch
 gomukhasana, 82, 128
Baddha konasana (butterfly), 75, 110, 114, 115, 124, 132, 133, 139
Bandha (energy locks), 52
 jalandhara, 53
 mula, 53
 uddiyana, 53
 'zip lock', 53
Bhujangasana, 66
Bidalasana (Cat Stretch), 83, 117, 132, 136
Boat (paripurna navasana), 74, 117, 138
Body brushing, 44
Body tone, 25
Body types, 18–21
 Ayurvedic, 18
 combinations, 18
 lean, 19
 muscular, 20
 round, 21
 somatyping, 18
Bones, 28
Bow (dhanurasana), 66, 117, 125, 126, 134
Brahmari, 51, 123
Breathing, 34–5
Breathing practices, 48–52
 alternate nostril breaths, 49
 agni sara (fire), 50, 114
 bandha, 52, 53
 brahmari (bee), 51, 123
 full Yogic breath, 50, 111, 123
 nadhi sodhana, 49, 111
 ohm, 52, 120, 129
 simhasana (lion), 52
 ujjayi (throat), 48, 114, 123, 132
Butterfly (baddha konasana), 75, 110, 111, 114, 115, 124, 132, 133, 139
Buttocks, slimming and toning, 130–9
Camel (ustrasana), 88, 89, 116, 117, 137
Cardiovascular fitness, 24, 146–7
Cat Stretch (bidalasana), 83, 117, 132, 136
Cellulite, 30

Chakra system, 113, 121–2, 130–1
 ajna, 122
 anahata, 121
 manipura, 113
 root, 131
 svadhisthana, 113
 visuddha, 122
Chandrasana (crescent moon), 87, 111, 116, 135
Chaturangasana (plank), 85, 145, 147
Chest, slimming and toning, 121–9
Child's Pose (supta vajrasana), 64, 116, 118, 126, 132, 135, 137, 143
Cobra, 66, 86, 126, 145
Cold or flu symptoms, 149
Cool-down session, 108
Corpse pose (savasana), 54, 111, 120, 129, 138
Cravings, 36
Crescent moon (chandrasana), 87, 111, 116, 135
Dancer (natarajasana), 101, 109, 128, 138
Dhanurasana (the bow), 66, 117, 125, 126, 134
Diabetes, 148
Diet, 40–4
 alkaline diet, 40, 42
 healthy recommendations, 41
 Yogic perspective, 40
Dog Stretch (adho mukha svanasana), 84, 118, 127, 133, 136, 143
Eka pada rajakapotasana (pigeon), 77, 132
Ectomorph, 18, 19
Endomorph, 18, 21
Endurance, 25
Energy seals, locks or directors see Bandha
Eye exercises, 79, 123
Face massage, 123
Fat, 30
 causes of excess fat, 30
 cellulite, 30
 good and bad, 43
 reducing fat deposits, 29
Fire breath (agni sara), 114
Fish (matsyana), 63, 124, 135
Fitness, 24, 25
 bones, 28
 metabolism, 29
Flexibility, 25
Full bridge (urdhva dhanurasana), 60, 126, 135
Gomukhasana, 82, 128
Guna, 40
Halasana (Plough), 62, 124, 135
Hatha Yoga

basic elements, 35
 endurance, 25–6
 physical fitness, 24, 25
 reducing fat deposits, 29
Head to knee pose (janu sirsasana), 70, 111, 114, 133
Heart
 aerobic exercise, 26
 medical condition, 148
High blood pressure, 148
Hips, slimming and toning, 130–9
Kapha body type, 18, 21
Kneeling postures, 82–9
 adho mukha svanasana (dog stretch), 84, 118, 127, 133, 136, 143
 bidalasana (cat stretch), 83, 117, 132, 136
 chandrasana (crescent moon), 87, 111, 116, 135
 chaturangasana (plank), 85, 145, 147
 push-up series, 86, 127
 supta vajrasana (child's pose), 82, 110, 118, 126, 132, 135, 137, 143
 ustrasana (camel), 88, 89, 116, 117, 137
 vasisthasana, 85
Kosha Yoga, 34
Ideal weight, 13
 how to achieve, 28
Janu sirsasana (head to knee), 70, 111, 114, 133
Jathara parivartanasana (spinal twists), 57, 119, 120, 129, 139
Legs, slimming and toning, 130–9
Lifestyle factors, 44
Lion breath (simhasana), 52, 123
Little bridge (setu bandha sarvangasana), 60, 115, 125, 134
Lock sets, 52, 53
Lower back
 mobilising exercises, 68, 114, 124, 133
 slimming and toning, 112–20
Lying postures, 54–67
 apanasana (wind-relieving), 55, 114, 115, 120, 125, 128, 133, 139
 bhujangasana, 66
 body curls, 65, 116, 125, 135
 cobra, 66, 86, 126, 145
 dhanurasana (bow), 66, 117, 125, 126, 134
 halasana (plough), 62, 124, 135
 jathara parivartanasana (spinal twists), 57, 119, 120, 129, 139
 leg raises, 58, 114, 125, 132
 leg walking, 59, 114, 132
 locust, 66
 matsyana (fish), 63, 124, 135
 rolling ball, 56, 115, 120, 124, 128, 134, 139

salabhasana, 66
sarvangasana, 61
savasana (corpse pose), 54, 111, 120, 129, 138
setu bandha sarvangasana (little bridge), 60, 115, 125, 134
shoulder stand, 61, 124, 134
sit-ups, 64, 116, 125, 135
urdhva dhanurasana (full bridge), 60, 126, 135
viparita karani, 61
Manipura chakra, 113
Massage, 44
Matsyana (fish), 63, 124, 135
Meditation, 48, 109, 111, 138
Menstruation, 105, 110, 143
Mesomorph, 18, 20
Metabolism, 29
Mobility, 25
Mountain pose (tadasana), 91, 92, 108, 109, 119, 126, 128, 129, 137, 138, 144, 146
Nadhi sodhana, 49, 111
Natarajasana (dancer), 101, 109, 128, 138
Neck stretches, 79, 115, 123
Obesity, 148
Ohm sound, 52, 120, 129
Overeating
  psychological factors, 34
Paripurna navasana, 74, 117, 138
Parivritta trikonsasana, 96
Pascimottanasana (sitting forward bend), 71, 111, 116–18, 124, 127, 133–6
Pigeon (eka pada rajakapotasana), 77, 132
Pitta body type, 18, 20
Plank (chaturangasana), 85, 86, 126, 145, 147
Plough (halasana), 62, 124, 135
Posture, 25
Postures, see Kneeling postures; Lying postures; Sitting postures; Standing postures
Pranayama (breathing practices), 48–52
Pregnancy, 148
  postnatal exercise, 149
Premenstrual tension relief, 110
Psychological health, 34–5, 112–13, 121–2, 130–1
  Kosha Yoga, 34
Push-ups, 86, 127
Rajasic diet, 40
Rolling ball, 56, 115, 120, 124, 128, 134, 139
Salabhasana, 66
Sanmukhi Mudra, 37
Sarvangasana, 61
Sattvic diet, 40
Savasana (corpse pose), 54, 111, 120,

129, 138
Setu bandha sarvangasana (little bridge), 60, 115, 125, 134
Shoulder Stand, 61, 124, 134
Simhasana (lion breath), 52, 123
Sitting postures, 68–79
  baddha konasana (butterfly), 75, 110, 114, 115, 124, 132, 133, 139
  crossed leg forward stretch, 78, 133
  eka pada rajakapotasana (pigeon), 77, 132
  half bridge, 72, 73, 127, 134, 135
  janu sirsasana (head to knee), 70, 111, 114, 133
  lower back mobilising, 68
  paripurna navasana (boat), 74, 117, 138
  pascimottanasana (sitting forward bend), 71, 111, 116–18, 124, 127, 133–6
  supta virasana, 78, 138
  upavista konasana (straddle), 76, 110, 114, 132
  upper body swing, 69, 114, 123
  vajrasana, 48, 109, 142
Sit-ups, 64, 116, 125, 135
Sleep, 44
Slimming and toning sessions, 104–139
  waistline and lower back, 112–20
  programme ideas, 106, 107
  short sessions, 108–111
  when to practise, 104
  where to practise, 104
Spinal twists (jathara parivartanasana), 57, 119, 120, 129, 139
Squat (utkatasana), 93, 127, 137
Standing postures, 90–101
  asymmetrical, counterpostures for, 100, 109, 126
  frog squat, 90, 136
  natarajasana (dancer), 101, 109, 138
  parivritta trikonsasana, 96
  parsva uttanasana, 108
  side bends, 92, 93, 119, 126
  spinal roll, 90, 118, 127, 136
  tadasana (mountain), 91, 92, 108, 109, 119, 126, 128, 129, 137, 138, 144, 146
  trikonasana (triangle), 95, 96, 119, 127, 136
  utkatasana (squat), 93, 127, 137
  uttanasana (standing forward bend), 94, 109, 111, 120, 127, 137
  virabhadrasana (warrior), 97, 98, 108, 119, 128, 136, 137
  vrksasana (tree), 101, 111, 119, 129, 138
  windmill versions, 99, 118
Straddle (upavista konasana), 76, 110, 114, 132
Strength, 25

Stress management, 36, 142–3
Sun salutations, 144–7
Supta vajrasana (Child's Pose), 82, 110, 116, 118, 126, 132, 135, 137, 143
Supta virasana, 78, 138
Svadhisthana chakra, 113
Tadasana (mountain), 91, 92, 108, 109, 119, 126, 128, 129, 137, 138, 144, 146
Tamasic diet, 40
Thyroid, 122
Tree pose (vrksasana), 101, 111, 119, 129, 138
Triangle pose (trikonasana), 95, 96, 119, 127, 136
Trikonsana (triangle), 95, 96, 119, 127, 136
Toning, 25
Touch techniques
  Sanmukhi Mudra, 37, 44
  Yoni, 37
Ujjayi breath, 48, 114, 123, 132
Upavista konasana (straddle), 76, 110, 114, 132
Upper body slimming and toning, 121–9
Urdhva dhanurasana (full bridge), 60, 126, 135
Ustrasana (camel), 88, 89, 116, 117, 137
Utkatasana (squat), 93, 127, 137
Uttanasana (standing forward bend), 94, 109, 111, 120, 127, 137
Vajrasana, 48, 109, 142
Vasisthasana, 85
Vinyasa, 140–7 see also Yoga flow
Viparita karani, 61
Virabhadrasana (warrior poses), 97, 98, 119, 128, 136, 137
Vitta body type, 18, 19
Vrksasana (tree), 101, 111, 119, 129, 138
Waistline, 112–20
Warm-up session, 108
Warrior poses (virabhadrasana), 97, 98, 108, 119, 128, 136, 137
Water, 43
Weight loss, 10–15
  diet, 40–4
  long-term solution to, 15
  unhealthy methods, 12
  water for, 43
  Yogic view, 10
Windmill exercises, 99, 118
Wind-relieving positions (apanasana), 55, 114, 115, 120, 125, 128, 129, 133, 139
Yoga flow, 140–7
  benefits, 140
  gentle, calming, soothing, 142–3
  sun salutations, 144–7
Yoni, 37